NEUROTRANSMITTER INTERACTIONS
IN THE BASAL GANGLIA

Neurotransmitter Interactions in the Basal Ganglia

Editors

M. Sandler, M.D.
Department of Chemical Pathology
Queen Charlotte's Maternity Hospital
London, United Kingdom

C. Feuerstein, M.D.
Laboratoire de Physiologie
Section Neurophysiologie
Pavillon de Neurologie
CHU de Grenoble
Grenoble Cedex, France

B. Scatton, Ph.D.
Laboratoires d'Etudes et de Recherches
Synthélabo (L.E.R.S.)
Bagneux, France

Raven Press ✍ New York

Raven Press, 1185 Avenue of the Americas, New York, New York 10036

Made in the United States of America

Library of Congress Cataloging-in-Publication Data

Neurotransmitter interactions in the basal
    ganglia.

    Includes bibliographies and index.
    1. Basal ganglia.   2. Neurotransmitters.
3. Neurotransmitter receptors.   I. Sandler,
Merton.   II. Feuerstein, C.   III. Scatton, B.
[DNLM: 1. Basal Ganglia—physiology.   2. Neuro-
regulators—physiology.   WL 307 N4947]
QP383.3.N48   1987   599'.0188   86-26157
ISBN 0-88167-267-X

The material contained in this volume was submitted as previously unpublished material, except in the instances in which credit has been given to the source from which some of the illustrative material was derived.

Papers or parts thereof have been used as camera-ready copy as submitted by the authors whenever possible; when retyped, they have been edited by the editorial staff only to the extent considered necessary for the assistance of an international readership. The views expressed and the general style adopted remain, however, the responsibility of the named authors. Great care has been taken to maintain the accuracy of the information contained in this volume. However, neither Raven Press nor the editors can be held responsible for errors or for any consequences arising from the use of the information contained herein.

Materials appearing in this book prepared by individuals as part of their official duties as U.S. Government employees are not covered by the above-mentioned copyright.

Authors were themselves responsible for obtaining the necessary permission to reproduce copyright material from other sources.

Preface

Unravelling the structure and function of the striatum has become a growth industry! Once the nigral lesion of Parkinson's disease had been identified and complemented by the seminal observation of Ehringer and Hornykiewicz of a striatal dopamine deficiency, the stage was set for a multidisciplinary onslaught on the basal ganglia. Neuroanatomists, neurophysiologists, neurologists, and psychiatrists all contributed to the information explosion that followed—and the new umbrella discipline of neuroscience was the beneficiary. One should never underestimate the importance of the L-dopa treatment of Parkinson's disease and the impetus it gave to these studies; yet it seems likely that the therapeutic benefit is actually achieved by a pharmacological trick. The basal ganglia and their connections are more subtle than that: dopamine remains of prime importance but many other neurotransmitters—acetylcholine, substance P, glutamate, enkephalins, to name but a few—are also vital for the normal functioning of this anatomical region. The whole situation is vastly more intricate than the pioneers of the 1970s ever imagined.

What has mainly changed, of course, is not only the availability of sophisticated new techniques but the realization that a multidisciplinary approach to the problems at hand is likely to yield the most handsome dividends. That it has done so is attested to by the harvest of new information gathered within these covers. We invited a group of world leaders from a number of different neuroscientific subdisciplines to contribute to this volume, and the resulting state of the art compilation is as exciting as it is topical. This book demonstrates how seemingly intractable problems can begin to yield before a combined interdisciplinary onslaught and cannot fail to be of interest and profit to neuroscientists of every orientation.

M. Sandler
C. Feuerstein
B. Scatton

Contents

Contributors

Luigi F. Agnati
Department of Human Physiology
University of Modena
Modena, Italy

S. Arbilla
Laboratoires d'Etudes et de Recherches
Synthélabo (L.E.R.S.)
58, rue de la Glacière
75013 Paris, France

G.W. Arbuthnott
MRC Brain Metabolism Unit
University Department of
* Pharmacology*
1 George Square
Edinburgh EH8 9JZ, United Kingdom

J. Artieda
Movement Disorders Unit
Neurology Department Clinica
* Universitaria*
University of Navarra Medical School
Pamplona 31080, Spain

G. Bartholini
Laboratoires d'Etudes et de Recherches
Synthélabo (L.E.R.S.)
58, rue de la Glacière
75013 Paris, France

Alain Beaudet
Laboratory of Neuroanatomy
Montreal Neurological Institute
3801 University Street
Montreal, Quebec, Canada H3A 2B4

S. Berrard
Laboratoire de Neurobiologie Cellulaire
* et Moléculaire*
Département de Génétique Moléculaire
CNRS
91190 Gif-Sur-Yvette, France

M.J. Besson
Chaire de Neuropharmacologie
INSERM U 114
Collège de France
11, place Marcelin Berthelot
75231 Paris Cedex 05, France

F. Blanot
Laboratoire de Neurobiologie Cellulaire
* et Moléculaire*
Département de Génétique Moléculaire
CNRS
91190 Gif-Sur-Yvette, France

J.P. Bolam
MRC Anatomical Neuropharmacology
* Unit*
Department of Pharmacology
South Parks Road
Oxford OX1 3QT, United Kingdom

C. Boni
Laboratoire de Neurobiologie Cellulaire
* et Moléculaire*
Département de Génétique Moléculaire
CNRS
91190 Gif-Sur-Yvette, France

J.R. Brown
Glaxo Research Group
Ware, United Kingdom

M. Buda
INSERM U 171 and CNRS LA 162
Hôpital Ste Eugénie
Pavillon 4H
69230 St. Genis Laval, France

A. Cheramy
Chaire de Neuropharmacologie
INSERM U 114
Collège de France
11, place Marcelin Berthelot
75231 Paris Cedex 05, France

G. Chevalier
Laboratoire des Neurosciences de la
Vision
Université Pierre et Marie Curie
4, place Jussieu
75230 Paris Cedex 05, France

A. Claudio Cuello
Department of Pharmacology and
Therapeutics
McGill University
3655 Drummond Street
Montreal, Quebec, Canada H3G 1Y6

J.M. Deminiere
Laboratoire de Physiologie des
Comportements Adaptatifs
INSERM U 259
Domaine de Carreire
rue Camille Saint-Saëns
33077 Bordeaux Cedex, France

J.M. Deniau
Laboratoire des Neurosciences de la
Vision
Université Pierre et Marie Curie
4, place Jussieu
75230 Paris Cedex 05, France

M. Desban
Chaire de Neuropharmacologie
INSERM U 114
Collège de France
11, place Marcelin Berthelot
75231 Paris Cedex 05, France

G. Di Chiara
Institute of Experimental Pharmacology
and Toxicology
University of Cagliari
Cagliari, Italy

N. Faucon Biguet
Laboratoire de Neurobiologie Cellulaire
et Moléculaire
Département de Génétique Moléculaire
CNRS
91190 Gif-Sur-Yvette, France

Kjell Fuxe
Department of Histology
Karolinska Institutet
Stockholm, Sweden

C. Gauchy
Chaire de Neuropharmacologie
INSERM U 114
Collège de France
11, place Marcelin Berthelot
75231 Paris Cedex 05, France

Charles F. Gerfen
Laboratory of Neurophysiology
National Institute of Mental Health
Bethesda, Maryland 20892

J.A. Girault
Chaire de Neuropharmacologie
INSERM U 114
Collège de France
11, place Marcelin Berthelot
75231 Paris Cedex 05, France

J. Glowinski
Chaire de Neuropharmacologie
INSERM U 114
Collège de France
11, place Marcelin Berthelot
75231 Paris Cedex 05, France

Menek Goldstein
Department of Psychiatry
New York University Medical Center
New York, New York 10016

F.G. Gonon
INSERM U 171 and CNRS LA 162
Hôpital Ste Eugénie
Pavillon 4H
69230 St. Genis Laval, France

B. Grima
Laboratoire de Neurobiologie Cellulaire
et Moléculaire
Département de Génétique Moléculaire
CNRS
91190 Gif-Sur-Yvette, France

Edith Hamel
Laboratory of Neuroanatomy
Montreal Neurological Institute
3801 University Street
Montreal, Quebec, Canada H3A 2B4

Anders Härfstrand
Department of Histology
Karolinska Institutet
Stockholm, Sweden

Ph. Horellou
*Laboratoire de Neurobiologie Cellulaire
et Moléculaire
Département de Génétique Moléculaire
CNRS
91190 Gif-Sur-Yvette, France*

A. Imperato
*Institute of Experimental Pharmacology
and Toxicology
University of Cagliari
Cagliari, Italy*

P.N. Izzo
*MRC Anatomical Neuropharmacology
Unit
Department of Pharmacology
South Parks Road
Oxford OX1 3QT, United Kingdom*

J.-F. Julien
*Laboratoire de Neurobiologie Cellulaire
et Moléculaire
Département de Génétique Moléculaire
CNRS
91190 Gif-Sur-Yvette, France*

M.L. Kemel
*Chaire de Neuropharmacologie
INSERM U 114
Collège de France
11, place Marcelin Berthelot
75231 Paris Cedex 05, France*

P.M. Laduron
*Department of Biochemical
Pharmacology
Janssen Pharmaceutica
B-2340 Beerse, Belgium*

A. Lamouroux
*Laboratoire de Neurobiologie Cellulaire
et Moléculaire
Département de Génétique Moléculaire
CNRS
91190 Gif-Sur-Yvette, France*

S.Z. Langer
*Laboratoires d'Etudes et de Recherches
Synthélabo (L.E.R.S.)
58, rue de la Glacière
75013 Paris, France*

M. Le Moal
*Laboratoire de Psychobiologie des
Comportements Adaptatifs
INSERM U 259
Domaine de Carreire
rue Camille Saint-Saëns
33077 Bordeaux Cedex, France*

A. Louilot
*Laboratoire de Psychobiologie des
Comportements Adaptatifs
INSERM U 259
Domaine de Carreire
rue Camille Saint-Saëns
33077 Bordeaux Cedex, France*

M.R. Luquin
*Movement Disorders Unit
Neurology Department Clinica
Universitaria
University of Navarra Medical School
Pamplona 31080, Spain*

N.K. MacLeod
*Department of Physiology
University of Edinburgh
Edinburgh, United Kingdom*

J. Mallet
*Laboratoire de Neurobiologie Cellulaire
et Moléculaire
Département de Génétique Moléculaire
CNRS
91190 Gif-Sur-Yvette, France*

F.M. Marcenac
*INSERM U 171 and CNRS LA 162
Hôpital Ste Eugénie
Pavillon 4H
69230 St. Genis Laval, France*

C.C. Mermet
*INSERM U 171 and CNRS LA 162
Hôpital Ste Eugénie
Pavillon 4H
69230 St. Genis Laval, France*

R. Mitchell
*MRC Brain Metabolism Unit
University Department of Pharmacology
1 George Square
Edinburgh EH8 9JZ, United Kingdom*

A. Mulas
*Institute of Experimental Pharmacology
and Toxicology
University of Cagliari
Cagliari, Italy*

Charles B. Nemeroff
*Department of Psychiatry and
Pharmacology
Duke University Medical Center
Durham, North Carolina 27710*

J.Z. Nowak
*Laboratoires d'Etudes et de Recherches
Synthélabo (L.E.R.S.)
58, rue de la Glacière
75013 Paris, France*

J.A. Obeso
*Movement Disorders Unit
Neurology Department Clinica
Universitaria
University of Navarra Medical School
Pamplona 31080, Spain*

Sven-Ove Ögren
*ASTRA Pharmaceuticals
Södertälje, Sweden*

J.M. Palacios
*Preclinical Research
SANDOZ Ltd.
CH-4002 Basle, Switzerland*

Emilio Merlo Pich
*Department of Human Physiology
University of Modena
Modena, Italy*

J. Powell
*Laboratoire de Neurobiologie Cellulaire
et Moléculaire
Département de Génétique Moléculaire
CNRS
91190 Gif-Sur-Yvette, France*

T. Rhyner
*Laboratoire de Neurobiologie Cellulaire
et Moléculaire
Département de Génétique Moléculaire
CNRS
91190 Gif-Sur-Yvette, France*

R. Romo
*Chaire de Neuropharmacologie
INSERM U 114
Collège de France
11, place Marcelin Berthelot
75231 Paris Cedex 05, France*

B. Scatton
*Laboratoires d'Etudes et de Recherches
Synthélabo (L.E.R.S.)
31, avenue Paul Vaillant Couturier
92220 Bagneux, France*

Wolfram Schultz
*Institut de Physiologie
Université de Fribourg
1700 Fribourg, Switzerland*

H. Simon
*Laboratoire de Psychobiologie des
Comportements Adaptatifs
INSERM U 259
Domaine de Carreire
rue Camille Saint-Saëns
33077 Bordeaux Cedex, France*

U. Spampinato
*Chaire de Neuropharmacologie
INSERM U 114
Collège de France
11, place Marcelin Berthelot
75231 Paris Cedex 05, France*

K. Taghzouti
*Laboratoire de Psychobiologie des
Comportements Adaptatifs
INSERM U 259
Domaine de Carreire
rue Camille Saint-Saëns
33077 Bordeaux Cedex, France*

K.H. Wiederhold
*Preclinical Research
SANDOZ Ltd.
CH-4002 Basle, Switzerland*

A.K. Wright
*MRC Brain Metabolism Unit
University Department of Pharmacology
1 George Square
Edinburgh EH8 9JZ, United Kingdom*

Isabella Zini
Department of Human Physiology
University of Modena
Modena, Italy

Michele Zoli
Department of Human Physiology
University of Modena
Modena, Italy

NEUROTRANSMITTER INTERACTIONS IN THE BASAL GANGLIA

Neurotransmitter Interactions in the Basal Ganglia, edited by M. Sandler et al.
Raven Press, New York © 1987.

FUNCTIONAL NEURONAL RELATIONS IN THE BASAL GANGLIA AND

THEIR CLINICAL RELEVANCE

G. Bartholini

Laboratoires d'Etudes et de Recherches Synthélabo (L.E.R.S.)
58, Rue de la Glacière, 75013, Paris

INTRODUCTION

Since the observation of the functional link between striatal dopamine (DA) and acetylcholine (ACh) neurons, numerous investigations have dealt with the interaction of neurotransmitters in the basal ganglia. The available data suggest the interplay of many more neuronal systems the functional meaning of which, however, still eludes our understanding. This paper therefore will focus on those aspects of neurotransmitter interaction which have clearly established clinical correlates, and thus which are most relevant to physiological and pathological function as well as to therapeutics. These neurotransmitters include DA, ACh and γ-aminobutyric acid (GABA); their function includes the regulation of extrapyramidal motility and muscle tone.

DA-ACh FUNCTIONAL LINK

In the early sixties McGeer and collaborators (15) hypothesized that a balance between catecholamines and ACh in the basal ganglia is essential for extrapyramidal function. Barbeau (1) modified this to the equilibrium between DA and ACh. This hypothesis - which was mainly based on the observation that both L-DOPA and anticholinergic agents ameliorate parkinsonian symptoms - was vague and remained so until the early seventies. At that time, perfusing the cat caudate nucleus under physiological conditions by means of an implanted push-pull cannula, and measurement of neurotransmitters in the perfusate, demonstrated that when dopaminergic transmission is blocked by neuroleptic agents, an increase in ACh liberation occurs (22). This is a result of DA receptor blockade which releases cholinergic interneurons from a tonic (12) inhibitory dopaminergic input, and is mediated by D_2 receptor subtypes as shown by Scatton (18). An opposite effect - a decrease in striatal ACh release - is obtained by electrical stimulation of the substantia nigra (6) or by administration of dopaminomimetics which enhances the inhibition of cholinergic interneurons (7, 22).

Behaviourally, the increase in cholinergic activity subsequent to reduction in DA-mediated transmission induces extrapyramidal symptoms, e.g. catalepsy in the rat, which are antagonized by anticholinergic agents (cfr. 7).

1

These experimental data support the hypothesis that some symptoms of Parkinson's disease and neuroleptic-induced parkinsonism are related to the enhanced activity of those cholinergic neurons which are released from the dopaminergic inhibition. The symptoms which depend on cholinergic hyperactivity are rigidity and possibly tremor. These respond not only to L-DOPA but also to anti-ACh compounds; in contrast, hypokinesia is ameliorated only by L-DOPA and does not appear therefore to be related to an enhanced cholinergic function (4).

The opposite mechanism, namely a decrease in cholinergic transmission, occurs under conditions of exaggerated DA receptor stimulation e.g. by dopaminomimetics or L-DOPA in parkinsonian patients exhibiting involuntary movements and in patients treated chronically with neuroleptics and suffering from tardive dyskinesia. The appearance of these symptoms is thought to be related to an enhancement of DA receptor density (23) in both conditions. An increased dopaminergic transmission and the subsequent reduction in cholinergic activity is supported by the fact that these involuntary movements are ameliorated by physostigmine and aggravated by anti-ACh agents (cfr. 10). Also, in the rat, choline acetyl transferase is reduced by chronic L-DOPA treatment (13) and a decrease in ACh release from the cat striatum is observed following repeated haloperidol administration (cfr. 2).

DA neuron activity is, conversely, influenced by ACh cells. The cholinergic input is of an excitatory nature as an increased cholinergic activity by oxotremorine, ACh and/or physostigmine enhances the release of DA from the cat caudate nucleus (3) whereas anticholinergic agents diminish DA turnover in the rat striatum (5). These data may be also relevant to the clinic ; they provide a sound explanation for the neurodysleptic syndrome occurring in some patients at the onset of the neuroleptic treatment, and which responds only to anti-ACh compounds : this syndrome is possibly triggered by an exaggerated DA liberation induced by cholinergic stimulation.

From the above data it appears that the DA-ACh-DA functional loop occupies a central place in the function of the basal ganglia inasmuch as its alterations induce major changes in extrapyramidal motility and muscle tone ; in this frame, the striatal cholinergic system translates changes of the nigro-striatal dopaminergic transmission into motor patterns.

INTERACTION OF GABA AND OTHER NEUROTRANSMITTERS

GABA-DA Functional Link

Another neurotransmitter which has been extensively investigated in the basal ganglia is GABA for which the available data are clinically relevant for extrapyramidal function. Striatal GABA neurons inhibit the activity of nigro-striatal DA cells by a double input, both at the cell bodies and the terminals. In agreement with electrophysiological results (cfr. 7) microinjection of GABA antagonists into the substantia nigra as well as into the striatum of the cat enhances DA turnover ; this effect is antagonized by GABA which by itself reduces the liberation of the amine. Similarly, systemic administration of GABA agonists reduces DA turnover (cfr. 4). Accordingly, the overall effect of GABA receptor stimulation results in a decreased dopaminergic activity ; this does not exclude that, in the substantia nigra, an inhibitory glycinergic interneuron is interposed between GABA terminals and DA cell bodies explaining the activation of DA neurons by GABA agonists observed under particular experimental conditions (9).

Also, the activation of the nigro-thalamic GABA path results in a behavioural syndrome similar to that induced by dopamino-mimetics ; however, this effect is not mediated by DA neurons but rather involves a cholinergic pathway (11).

GABA-ACh Functional Link

In the striatum, GABA neurons exert an inhibitory influence on cholinergic interneurons. Thus, in the rat, GABA mimetics enhance ACh concentrations (which reflects a decreased turnover of the neurotransmitter), antagonize the neuroleptic-induced reduction in ACh levels and decrease the hemicholinium-3-induced ACh disappearance (20 ; see also B. Scatton, this Symposium). The reduction in striatal ACh turnover by GABA agonists occurs at about $^1/_{10}$ of the threshold dose which reduces DA neuron activity (21).

The GABA input on striatal cholinergic neurons is probably indirect. Thus, when cortico-striatal afferents are sectioned, GABA agonists no longer reduce striatal ACh turnover (19). It appears therefore that GABA neurons inhibit a cortico-striatal path which provides an excitatory input to cholinergic interneurons ; this path is probably glutamatergic in nature as previously demonstrated (16).

Clinical implications of the GABA-DA-ACh Link. Apart from the results of local injections of GABA agonists or antagonists into discrete brain areas (see above), there is no evidence in the normal state for major behavioural changes induced by GABA mimetics. Maybe, under physiological conditions, GABA-mediated inhibition is already maximal or powerful homeostatic mechanisms counterbalance the changes induced by the increased GABAergic transmission. However, when GABA mimetics are combined with other drugs which alter neurotransmission, then behavioural effects occur. Clearcut examples are the interactions of GABA agonists with neuroleptics and dopaminomimetics. Thus, the cataleptogenic action of neuroleptics is antagonized by coadministration of low doses of GABA agonists ; higher doses of these drugs potentiate the neuroleptic-induced catalepsy (25). While the effect of high doses of GABA mimetics can be attributed to reduced DA release - which enhances the effect of DA receptor blockade - the effect of low doses is probably due to inhibition of striatal cholinergic neurons which results in a facilitation of the effect of DA receptor stimulation (see above).

Opposite effects are observed when GABA agonists are combined with dopaminomimetics : low doses of GABA agonists potentiate stereotypies induced by apomorphine probably via inhibition of cholinergic neurons ; higher doses antagonize apomorphine (24). This latter effect results from an unknown GABAergic mechanism which probably takes place beyond the DA receptor and which tunes the effect of an exaggerated DA receptor stimulation (14).

From these data in animals, it can be expected that moderate doses of GABA receptor agonists - owing to their specific inhibition of ACh interneurons - would improve parkinsonian symptoms with a possible aggravation of L-DOPA induced involuntary movements ; these effects have indeed been reported (8). Conversely, higher doses - by reducing DA turnover and by modulating postsynaptically the effects of DA receptor stimulation - should improve tardive dyskinesia. This hypothesis has been confirmed by open and double blind studies in schizophrenic patients (17).

CONCLUSION

From the data discussed in this review, it appears that DA, ACh, GABA and probably glutamate neurons play a fundamental role in the basal ganglia under physiological and pathological conditions.

Alteration of the complex interactions of these neurons leads to major behavioural changes as indicated in animals and humans by the effects of agonists and antagonists. It has however to be kept in mind that, although there is an astonishing convergence of experimental, clinical and therapeutic data, the interaction models which have been discussed are, by definition, oversimplified as they do not take into consideration other components such as 5-HT, enkephalines, substance P etc. However, no evidence is provided as yet that the alteration of the function of these latter transmitters leads to such major behavioural changes as described for the DA, ACh and GABA systems.

REFERENCES

1. Barbeau, A. (1962): Canad. med. Ass. J., 87:802-807.
2. Bartholini, G. and Lloyd, K.G. (1980): In: Handbook of Experimental Pharmacology: Psychotropic Agents : Antipsychotics and Antidepressants, edited by F. Hoffmeister and G. Stille, pp. 193-212, Springer-Verlag, Heidelberg.
3. Bartholini, G. and Stadler, H. (1975): In: Chemical Tools in Catecholamine Research, edited by O. Almgren, A. Carlsson and J. Engel, pp. 235-241, North Holland Publishing Co., Amsterdam.
4. Bartholini, G. and Stadler, H. (1976): In: Advances in Parkinsonism, edited by W. Birkmeyer and O. Hornykiewicz, pp. 115-123, Editiones Roche, Basle.

5. Bartholini, G., Keller, H. H. and Pletscher, A. (1975): J. of Pharmacy and Pharmacology, 27:439-442.
6. Bartholini, G., Stadler, H., Gadea-Ciria, M., and Lloyd, K.G. (1975): In: Antipsychotic Drugs. Pharmacodynamics & Pharmacokinetics, edited by G. Sedvall, pp. 105-116, Pergamon Press, Oxford.
7. Bartholini, G., Stadler, H., Gadea-Ciria, M. and Lloyd, K.G. (1976): Neuropharmacology, 15:515-519.
8. Bergman, K.J., Limongi, J.C.P., Lowe, Y.H., Mendoza, M.R. and Yahr, M.D. (1984): Lancet 1(8376):559.
9. Cheramy, A., Nieoullon, A. and Glowinski, J. (1978): Eur. J. Pharmacol., 48:281-295.
10. Davis, K.L., Hollister, L.E., Berger, P.A. and Barchas, J.D. (1975): Psychopharmacol. Commun., 1:533-543.
11. Di Chiara, G., Porceddu, M.L., Morelli, M., Mulas, M.L. and Gessa, G.L. (1978): In: GABA-Neurotransmitters edited by H. Kofod, J. Scheel-Krüger and P. Krogsgaard-Larsen, pp. 465-481, Munksgaard, Copenhagen.
12. Guyenet, P.G., Agid, Y., Javoy, J., Beaujouan, J.C., Rossier, J. and Glowinski, J. (1975): Brain Res., 84:227-244.
13. Lloyd, K.G. and Hornykiewicz, O. (1977): Life Sci., 21:1489-1496.
14. Lloyd, K.G., Broekkamp, C.L. and Worms, P. (1983): In: Applications of Behavioural Pharmacology in Toxicology, edited by G. Zbinden, V. Cuomo, G. Racagni and B. Weiss, pp. 203-215, Raven Press, New York.
15. McGeer, P.L., Boulding, J.E., Gibson, W.C., Foulkes, R.G., (1961): JAMA 177:665-670.
16 McGeer, P.L., McGeer, E.G., Scherer, V. and Singh, K. (1977): Brain Res., 128:369-373.
17. Morselli, P.L., Fournier, V. Bossi, L. and Musch, B. (1985): In: Dyskinesia Research and Treatment, edited by D. Casey, T.N. Chase, A.V. Christensen and J. Gerlach, pp. 128-136, Springer Verlag, Heidelberg.
18. Scatton, B. (1982): Life Sci., 31:2883-2890.
19. Scatton, B. and Bartholini, G. (1980): Brain Res., 200:174-178.
20. Scatton, B. and Bartholini, G. (1982): J. Pharmacol. Exp. Ther., 220:689-695.
21. Scatton, B., Zivkovic, B., Dedek, J., Lloyd, K.G., Constantinidis, J., Tissot, R. and Bartholini, G. (1982): J. Pharmacol. Exp. Ther., 220:678-688.
22. Stadler, H., Lloyd, K.G., Gadea-Cirea, M. and Bartholini, G. (1973): Brain Res., 55:476-480.
23. Tarsy, D. and Baldessarini, R.J. (1977): Biol. Psychiat., 12:431-450.
24. Worms, P., Depoortere, H., Durand, A., Morselli, P.L., Lloyd, K.G. and Bartholini, G. (1982): J. Pharmacol. Exp. Ther. 220:660-671.
25. Worms, P. and Lloyd, K.G. (1980): Naunyn-Schmiedeberg's Arch. Pharmacol., 311:179-184.

Neurotransmitter Interactions in the Basal Ganglia, edited by M. Sandler et al.
Raven Press, New York © 1987.

CHOLINERGIC COMPONENTS OF THE BASAL GANGLIA

A. Claudio Cuello

Department of Pharmacology and Therapeutics, McGill
University, 3655 Drummond Street, Montreal, Quebec, H3G 1Y6

Identification of cholinergic neurons in the CNS

The possibility that acetylcholine could play a major
neurotransmitter role in the CNS was advanced early in this
century by Chang and Gaddum, Feldberg and Vogt, MacIntosh
and others (6, 14, 23, 11). Despite the evidence provided
with biochemical and pharmacological approaches of the time,
it was exceedingly difficult for decades to relate the
biosynthesis and release of acetylcholine to defined CNS
neuronal systems. This was also in contrast with the well
resolved problem of   cholinergic involvement in
peripheral motor and sympathetic neurons. CNS cholinergic
neurons remained elusive to anatomical identification due to
the lack of a proper histochemical procedure to detect
acetylcholine. Important attempts at defining these
presumptive CNS cholinergic systems were made by many
authors applying histochemical procedures for the
demonstration of the inactivating enzyme acetyl
cholinesterase (AChE). The work of Shute and Lewis has been
fundamental in alerting us to the existence of possible
cholinergic cell groups and pathways (33, 22). Nevertheless,
even before immunocytochemistry resolved the problem of
specificity, it became clear that not all AChE reactive
neurons were necessarily truly cholinergic. This has been
well illustrated by Butcher and collaborators in the case of
the dopaminergic neurons of the substantia nigra (5). The
more convincing definition of central cholinergic neurons
awaited the introduction of immunocytochemistry (ICC)
demonstrating sites containing the acetylcholine
biosynthetic enzyme (choline acetyltransferase, usually
referred to as ChAT or CAT). This approach was pioneered by
Kimura and collaborators (19) and, soon after, Eckenstein,
Barde and Thoenen (12) produced very specific antibodies
against the highly purified preparations of the enzyme,
which met the criteria set by the most critical observers
(see reference 30). Since then, several laboratories have
reported the development of monoclonal antibodies to ChAT
and their successful application for the immunocytochemical
demonstration of CNS cholinergic neurons. Thanks to these
tools, a picture of the CNS distribution of ChAT
immunoreactive cell bodies, terminals and pathways is

steadily emerging (for reviews see 15, 8, 34, 28). Here we
will refer to aspects of cholinergic neurons found within
the boundaries of the corpus striatum of the rat (globus
pallidus and caudate-putamen).

<u>Cholinergic neurons in the basal ganglia</u>

     The most prominent cholinergic components of the basal
ganglia are in the caudate-putamen and innermost portions of
the globus pallidus. ChAT immunoreactive neurons are also
found in the nucleus accumbens and ventral striatum (see
Fig. 1).

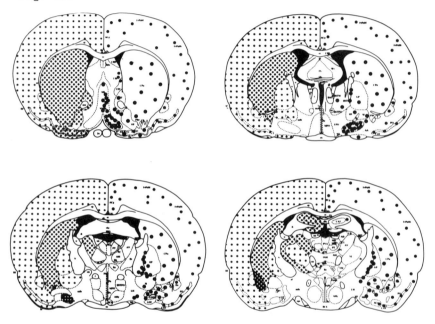

Fig. 1. Schematic representation of the distribution and
relative abundance of ChAT immunoreactive cell bodies (large
dots, right side) and fibers and nerve terminals (small
dots, left side) in the forebrain components of the basal
ganglia of the rat. From Sofroniew et al (34).

     In order to establish how this anatomical
compartmentalization corresponds with cholinergic
biochemical parameters we have assayed, following the
procedure of Fonnum (16), the ChAT activity in
microdissected samples of the corpus striatum. Thus, we have
separately analyzed those regions of the globus pallidus
containing cholinergic cell bodies from those which only

contain a loose network of processes (see Table 1). The results obtained showed a good correlation with ICC. In addition, they indicated that a considerable amount of ChAT activity was present in axonal processes located in regions of the globus pallidus which are devoid of cholinergic cell bodies. As neostriatal cholinergic neurons do not seem to project to the globus pallidus (see below), the most likely origin of this contingent is the nucleus basalis magnocellularis (NBM).

Table 1

Choline acetyltransferase (ChAT) enzymatic activity in the micro-dissected nucleus basalis magnocellularis, globus pallidus (including & excluding area of n.b.m.) and caudate-putamen of the rat

	ChAT n.moles/mg protein/h	n
n. basalis m. (NBM)	53.3 ± 3.2	5
globus pallidus (excluding NBM)	38.1 ± 3.2	4
(including NBM)	60.5 ± 6.1	4
caudate putamen	120.5 ± 5.5	5

Values represent the mean ± the standard error of the mean. n = number of cases

Caudate-putamen

The ChAT immunoreactive neurons of the caudate-putamen are large (18-25 μm diameter, according to Sofroniew et al (34), 20-44 μm diameter, according to Paxinos and Butcher (28)). They are multipolar elements with long dendrites. They have been identified as medium to large aspiny or sparsely spiny neurons (19, 17, 3). They probably constitute 1 to 3 percent of the neuronal population of the nucleus (40). They are responsible for the rich ChAT immunoreactive, and partly for the AChE positive network of the neostriatum. These neurons most probably do not project axonal arborizations beyond the caudate-putamen. The intrinsic (local circuit) nature of these cells is supported by studies combining tract tracing techniques with AChE histochemistry (17, 40, 27). In view of the considerable ChAT activity detected in the globus pallidus in areas devoid of cholinergic cell bodies, we reinvestigated this problem by combining tract tracing techniques with ChAT immunocytochemistry. For this, we stereotaxically injected 0.1 and 0.2 µl of 20% horseradish peroxidase (HRP) in the globus pallidus. To prevent non-specific incorporation of the marker and needle damage, we penetrated the brain at an angle from the contralateral side. Out of a series of 19 rats, we selected the three best cases for ICC. In all the three cases, a large number of caudate-putamen neurons retrogradely transported HRP, but none of these neurons displayed ChAT immunoreactivity (see Fig. 2). Thus, the pallidal cholinergic compartment is anatomically and, presumably, functionally independent of the neostriatal cholinergic compartment.

Globus pallidus

The globus pallidus in the rat contains a large number of cholinergic neurons of analogous dimensions from those observed in the caudate-putamen. These neurons occupy the innermost portions of the globus pallidus and invade the adjacent capsula interna. This cholinergic group spread over two-thirds of the rat globus pallidus at most caudal levels. This group is probably continued with cholinergic cells of the ventral striatum and with scattered cells found in the anterior hypothalamus (8, 15, 17, 18, 24, 27, 32, 34, 40, 41). The ensemble has been referred to as a Ch4 group by Mesulam and coworkers (24). That these neurons project widely to the cerebral cortex has been envisaged from earlier works of Shute and Lewis (33) and Krnjevic and Silver (20), and confirmed more recently combining tract tracing techniques with ICC (41, 36, 32).

Cortical-n. basalis relationships

Besides the widespread cholinergic supply to the cerebral cortex, the NBM receives reciprocal input from the cerebral cortex, the extent of which, and the differences among species, are being studied in several laboratories. It is also clear that the cortex contains an intrinsic component which accounts for about 30% of the total neuronal cholinergic population of the cerebral cortex (21, 7) (see Fig. 1). A decrease of cholinergic markers in the cerebral cortex has been demonstrated in cases of Alzheimer's disease (4, 10). This cortical cholinergic deficit has been attributed to cell losses in the NBM (38) and suggested to be a primary cause for clinical manifestations. There is

nevertheless some discrepancy as to whether these cells are
indeed lost in advanced cases (30), reduced in number
moderately (25), or present in a shrunken state (29). In
order to test whether the involvement of cholinergic neurons
of NBM in Alzheimer's disease is a primary or secondary
consequence of cortical damage, a rat model was developed by
Sofroniew and collaborators (34). In this model, extensive
cortical damage revealed swollen ChAT immunoreactive neurons
in the NBM ipsilateral to the lesion, initially, and shrunk
cells with fewer processes, at later stages (32, 36, 84, 120
days) (34). Interestingly enough, the number of cells
remained unchanged in these experiments.

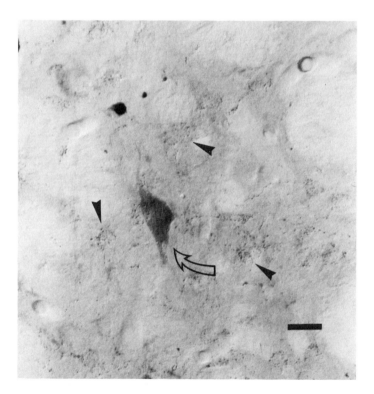

Fig. 2. Combined retrograde tracing of horseradish
peroxidase implanted in the globus pallidus and ChAT
immunostaining. Note that a large number of caudate putamen
neurones have retrogradely transported the tracer (filled
arrows). In the center of the field a large ChAT
immunoreactive neuron free of tracer can be observed (open
arrow). Interference optic. Scale bar=25 µm.

Further to this, we have investigated the biochemical correlates of these changes and have noticed that a parallel decrease in ChAT activity occurs in microdissected samples of the NBM, while glutamic acid decarboxylase activity (GAD) remained at control levels (see reference 35) (see Table 2). None of the other areas studied (n. accumbens, amygdala, hippocampus, caudate-putamen, septum) showed alterations in the enzymatic activity of ChAT or GAD. In this series where young animals were utilized, a recovery on NBM ChAT activity was noticed at 120 days following cortical lesions (see Table 2).

Table 2

ChAT activity in microdissected nucleus basalis of the rat in control animals and following unilateral (left) decortication

Time	ChAT activity nmol/mg protein/h	SEM	n	Percent of control
Nucleus basalis				
Control	51.9	1.8	33	--
10-day left	39.9	5.6	6	76.7*
right	49.0	4.9		94.4
30-day left	41.0	4.8	6	70.0*
right	42.5	3.2		81.9*
80-day left	38.2	3.4	4	73.6*
right	47.3	5.6		91.1
120-day left	48.4	3.5	5	93.3
right	50.1	4.3		96.5

Values represent the means ± SEM n, Number of samples. * $p < 0.05$, Student t test.   From reference (35).

A similar spontaneous recovery on ChAT activity has been noticed in the cerebral cortex of the rat after intrapallidal injections of ibotenic acid (37). In subsequent studies, we observed that no recovery in ChAT activity takes place in the NBM of aged animals following cortical damage (Stephens, Tagari and Cuello, unpublished). These observations might have some bearing on retrograde neurodegenerative disorders, including Alzheimer's disease. There is evidence that regenerative changes can take place in the mammalian nervous system following injury (2, 26) and that endogenous factors contribute to it. Amongst these endogenous factors are the sialogangliosides which can reduce neuronal damage and promote regeneration in the CNS (1, 39). With this in mind, we have attempted the prevention of these changes by the chronic application of the ganglioside GM1. The chronic intraperitoneal application of GM1 (Fidia) (30mg/kg daily) completely prevented the ipsilateral cell shrinkage of NBM ChAT immunoreactive neurons as well as the otherwise observed depletion of ChAT activity in the area (9).

In these experiments, we have also observed an increment of ChAT activity in the NBM of GM1 treated, sham operated animals. The protective effects of GM1 on the retrograde neurodegenerative changes of cholinergic neurons of the NBM did not extend to aged animals under similar experimental conditions (Stephens, Tagari, Cuello, unpublished).

Conclusions

The cholinergic cells of the caudate-putamen are a key element in the local circuitry of the nucleus. Tract tracing combined with immunocytochemistry indicate that these cells do not project beyond the limits of the caudate-putamen. The cholinergic innervation of the globus pallidus in the rat is seemingly derived from cell bodies belonging to the rodent equivalent of the nucleus basalis. The cholinergic neurons of the nucleus basalis should be considered an integral part of the basal ganglia, at least in the rat. The morphology and biochemistry of this population of cholinergic neurons is dependent on the integrity of the cerebral cortex. Lesions of the cerebral cortex in the rat produces cell shrinkage and loss of dendritic profiles and specific depletion of ChAT activity, but not change in GAD activity. In young animals, these biochemical-anatomical changes can be prevented by the chronic administration of sialogangliosides.

Acknowledgements

I wish to thank Mr. A. Forster for his photographic work and Mrs. S. MacMillan for her skillfull secretarial assistance. Grant support is acknowledged from the Medical Research Council of Canada and also from the Office of the Dean of Medicine, McGill University. The monoclonal antibody against ChAT was a gift of Boehringer.

References

1.   Agnati, L.F., Fuxe, K., Calza, L., Benfenati, F., Cavicchioli, L., Toffano, G., and Goldstein, M. (1983) Gangliosides increase the survival of lesioned dopamine neurons and favour the recovery of dopaminergic synaptic function in striatum of rats by collateral sprouting. Acta Phys. Scand. 119: 347-363.

2.   Bjorklund, A., and Stenevi, U. (1979) Regeneration of monoaminergic and cholinergic neurons in the mammalian central nervous system. Physiol. Rev. 59: 62-100.

3.   Bolam, J.P., Ingham, C.A., and Smith, A.D. (1984). The section-Golgi-impregnation procedure-3. Combination of Golgi-impregnation with enzyme histochemistry and electron microscopy to characterize acetylcholinesterase-containing neurones in the rat neostriatum. Neuroscience 12: 687-709.

4.   Bowen, D.M., Smith, C.B., White, P., and Davidson, A.N. (1976). Neurotransmitter related enzymes and indices of hypoxia in senile dementia and other abiotrophies. Brain 99: 459-496.

5.   Butcher, L.L., and Marchand, R. (1978) Dopamine neurons in pars compacta of the substantia nigra contain acetylcholinesterase: Histochemical correlations of the same brain section. Eur. J. Pharmacol. 52: 415-417.

6.   Chang H.C. and Gaddum J.H. (1933) Choline esters in tissue extracts. J. Physiol. (Lond.) 79: 255-285.

7.   Coyle, J.T., and Schwarcz, R. (1983) The use of excitatory amino acids as selective neurotoxins. In A. Bjorklund and T. Hokfelt (Eds.) Handbook of Chemical Neuroanatomy. Vol. 1: Methods in Chemical Neuroanatomy. Elsevier, Amsterdam, pp. 508-527.

8.   Cuello, A.C., and Sofroniew, M.V. (1984) The anatomy of the CNS cholinergic neurons. Trends in NeuroSciences 7: 74-78.

9.   Cuello, A.C., Stephens, P.H., Tagari, P.C., Sofroniew, M.V. and Pearson, R.C.A. (1986) Retrograde changes in the nucleus basalis of the rat, caused by cortical damage, are prevented by exogenous ganglioside GM1. Brain Res. (in press).

10.   Davies, P. and Moloney, A.J.F. (1976) Selective losses of central cholinergic neurones in Alzheimer's disease. Lancet ii: 143.

11.   Dikshit, B.B. (1934) Action of acetylcholine on the brain and its occurrence therein. J. Physiol. (Lond.) 80: 409-421.

12.   Eckenstein, F., Barde, Y.A., and Thoenen, H. (1981) Production of cholinergic innervation in cortex, one co-localized with vasoactive intestinal polypeptide. Nature 309: 153-155.

13. Feldberg, W. (1945) Present views on the mode of action of acetylcholine in the central nervous system. Physiol. Rev. 25: 596-642.

14. Feldberg, W., and Vogt, M. (1948) Acetylcholine synthesis in different regions of the central nervous system. J. Physiol. (Lond.) 107: 372-381.

15. Fibiger, H.C. (1982) The organization and some projections of cholinergic neurons of the mammalian forebrain. Brain Res. Rev. 4: 327-388.

16. Fonnum, F. (1975) A rapid radiochemical method for the determination of choline acetyltransferase. J. Neurochem. 24: 407-409.

17. Henderson, Z. (1981) Ultrastructure and acetylcholinesterase content of neurones forming connections between the striatum and substantia nigra of the rat. J. Comp. Neurol. 197: 185-196.

18. Ingham, C.A., Bolam, J.P., Wainer, B.H., and Smith, A.D. (1985) A correlated light and electron microscopic study of identified cholinergic basal forebrain neurons that project to the cortex in the rat. J. Comp. Neurol. 239: 176-192.

19. Kimura, H., McGeer, P.L., Peng, F., and McGeer, E.G. (1980) Choline acetyltransferase-containing neurons in rodent brain demonstrated by immunohistochemistry. Science 208: 1057-1059.

20. Krnjevic, K., and Silver, A. (1965) A histochemical study of cholinergic fibers in the cerebral cortex. J. Anat. 99: 711-759.

21. Lehman, J., Nagy, J.I., Atmadja, S., and Fibiger, H.C. (1980) The nucleus basalis magnocellularis: the origin of a cholinergic projection to the neocortex of the rat. Neuroscience 5: 1161-1174.

22. Lewis, P.R., and Shute, C.C.D. (1967) The cholinergic limbic system: projections to hippocampal formation, medial cortex, nuclei of the ascending cholinergic reticular system, and subfornical organ and supraoptic crest. Brain 90: 521-542.

23. MacIntosh, F.C. (1941) The distribution of acetylcholine in the peripheral and the central nervous system. J. Physiol. (Lond.) 99: 436-442.

24. Mesulam, M.M., Mufson, E.J., Wainer, B.H., and Levey, A.I. (1983) Central cholinergic pathways in the rat: an overview based on alternative nomenclature (Ch1-Ch6). Neuroscience 10: 1185-1201.

25. Nagai, T., McGeer, P.L., Peng, E.G., and Dolman, C.E. (1983) Choline acetyltransferase immunohistochemistry in brains of Alzheimer's disease patients and controls. Neurosci. Lett. 36: 195-199.

26. Nicholls, J.G. (Ed.) (1982) Repair and regeneration of
     the nervous system. Life Sciences Research Report 24:
     Springer-Verlag (Berlin/Heidelberg/New York).
27. Parent, A., Boucher, R. and O'Reilly-Fromentin, J.
     (1981). Acetylcholinesterase-containing neurons in cat
     pallidal complex: Morphological characteristics and
     projection towards the neocortex. Brain Res. 230: 356-
     361.
28. Paxinos, G., and Butcher, L.L. (1985) Organizational
     principles of the brain as revealed by choline
     acetyltransferase and acetylcholinesterase distribution
     and projections. In G. Paxinos (Ed.) The Rat Nervous
     System. Academic Press, Sydney, pp. 487-521.
29. Pearson, R.C.A., Sofroniew, M.V., Cuello, A.C., Powell,
     T.P.S., Eckenstein, F., Esiri, M.M., and Wilcock, G.K.
     (1983) Persistence of cholinergic neurons in the basal
     nucleus in a brain with senile dementia of the
     Alzheimer's type demonstrated by immunohistochemical
     staining for choline acetyltransferase. Brain Res. 289:
     375-379.
30. Perry, R.H., Candy, J.M., Perry, E.K., Irving, D.,
     Blessed, G., Fairbairn, A.F., and Tomlinson, B.E.
     (1982) Neurosci. Lett. 33: 311-313.
31. Rossier, J. (1981) Serum monospecificity: a
     prerequisite for reliable immunohistochemical
     localization of neuronal markers including choline
     acetyltransferase. Neuroscience 6: 989-991.
32. Rye, D.B., Mesulam, M.M., Mufson, E.J., Saper, C.B.,
     and Wainer, B.H. (1984) Cortical projections arising
     from the basal forebrain: A study of cholinergic versus
     non-cholinergic components employing combined
     retrograde tracing and immunohistochemical localization
     of choline acetyltransferase. Neuroscience 13: 627-
     643.
33. Shute, C.C.D., and Lewis, P.R. (1967) The ascending
     cholinergic reticular system: neocortical, olfactory
     and subcortical projections. Brain 90: 497-520.
34. Sofroniew, M.V., Eckenstein, F., and Cuello, A.C.
     (1985a) Central cholinergic neurons visualized by
     immunohistochemical detection of choline
     acetyltransferase. In G. Paxinos and C. Watson (Eds.)
     The Rat Nervous System. Academic Press, Sydney,
35. Stephens, P.H., Cuello, A.C., Sofroniew, M.V., Pearson,
     R.C.A., and Tagari, P. (1985) The effects of unilateral
     decortication upon choline acetyltransferase and
     glutamate decarboxylase activities in the nucleus
     basalis and other areas of the rat brain. J.
     Neurochem. 45: 1021-1026.

36. Wainer, B.H., and Rye, D.B. (1984) Retrograde
     horseradish peroxidase tracing combined with the
     localization of choline acetyltransferase
     immunoreactivity. J. Histochem. Cytochem. 32: 439-443.
37. Wenk, G.L., and Olton, D.S. (1984) Recovery of
     neocortical ChAT activity following ibotenic acid
     injection into the nucleus basalis of Meynert in rats.
     Brain Res. 293: 184-186.
38. Whitehouse, P.J., Price, D.L., Struble, R.G., Clark,
     A.W., Coyle, J.T. and De Long, M.R. (1982) Alzheimer's
     disease and senile dementia loss of neurons in the
     basal forebrain. Science 215: 1237-1239.
39. Wojcik, M., Ulas, J., and Oderfeld-Nowak, B. (1982) The
     stimulating effect of ganglioside injections on the
     recovery of choline acetyltransferase activities in the
     hippocampus of the rat after septal lesions.
     Neuroscience 7: 494-499.
40. Woolf, N.J., and Butcher. L.L. (1981). Cholinergic
     neurons in the caudate-putamen complex proper are
     intrinsically organized: A combined Evans Blue and
     acetylcholinesterase analysis. Brain Res. Bull. 7: 487-
     507.
41. Woolf, N.J., Eckenstein, F., and Butcher, L.L. (1983)
     Cholinergic projections from the basal forebrain to the
     frontal cortex: A combined fluorescent tracer and
     immunohistochemical analysis in the rat. Neurosci.
     Lett. 40: 93-98.

Neurotransmitter Interactions in the Basal Ganglia, edited by M. Sandler et al.
Raven Press, New York © 1987.

THE NEOSTRIATAL MOSAIC:

THE REITERATED PROCESSING UNIT

Charles R. Gerfen

Laboratory of Neurophysiology,
National Institute of Mental Health,
Bethesda, Maryland, 20892

Receiving inputs from the majority of the cerebral cortex, the neostriatum functions to affect virtually all aspects of behavior. Not only does the striatum, as a major part of the basal ganglia, regulate such diverse fuctions as movement, mood and memory (8) but the complex clinical disorders that accompany basal ganglia dysfunction suggest that these functions are normally integrated by this neural system. Recent studies provide insights as to how the neuroanatomical and neurochemical systems of the basal ganglia, and the neostriatum in particular, are organized to accomplish such integration. Dual organizational schemes exist in striatal connections. In one scheme certain input and output pathways of the striatum are topographically ordered, which conveys a degree of regional specialization to different striatal areas. For example, the dorsal striatum receives inputs from sensorimotor cortical areas (among other areas) and projects to the substantia nigra pars reticulata, whereas the ventral striatum receives inputs from limbic brain areas such as the olfactory cortex, amygdala and hippocampus and projects to the substantia nigra pars compacta (21, 26,31). In the other scheme there is a divergence of both corticostriate (15, 37,40) and striatonigral (11) projection systems. The consequent overlap in these afferent systems results first in the convergence at each striatal locus of inputs from multiple, widespread cortical areas and a subsequent convergence onto each locus in the substantia nigra of inputs from widespread striatal areas. This duality of organizational schemes provides for the maintenance of topographic order in systems such as those providing movement and sensory inputs into the system (4, 30), and allows for interaction in the striatum between inputs from regionally separated cortical areas. Recent studies suggest that the neurochemical compartmentation of the striatum reflects the existence of a reiterated system of local processing units distributed throughout the striatum that impart some common rules to the manner of interaction of cortical inputs with output systems of the striatum (9,11).

COMPARTMENTAL ORGANIZATION OF THE NEOSTRIATUM

Nissl stained sections show a homogenous distribution of striatal neurons that masks the compartmental organization of the
striatum revealed with the localization of neurochemical markers
(12,18,22,34). Two striatal compartments, the patch and matrix,
form a mosaic throughout the striatum. Figure 1 shows adjacent
coronal sections through the rat striatum reacted to reveal the
relationship of the patch compartment, marked in A with 3H-Nalox-
one binding to mu opiate receptor sites (22,34) and the matrix,
marked in B with calcium binding protein (CaBP) immunoreactivity
(12). The complementary distribution of these two markers is
maintained throughout the striatum and thus defines the patch-
matrix compartmental organization of the striatum. Other neurochemical markers, such as somatostatin-fiber immunoreactivity
(9,11) and acetylcholinesterase (AChE) histochemical staining
(18,22) also mark the matrix compartment. Not all striatal
neurochemical systems are selectively distributed according to
patch-matrix patterns. Dopaminergic afferents are evenly distributed throughout the striatum (32) and peptides such as substance P, enkephalin and dynorphin show a mixed pattern, being
concentrated in patches in some striatal areas while in other
areas being distributed in both compartments (17,19,27). However, as will be discussed below, the connections of such
neurochemical systems are compartmentalized.

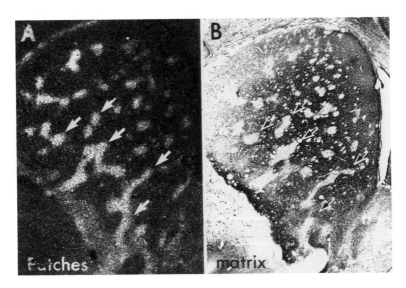

FIG. 1. A) 3H-Naloxone binding of mu opiate receptors to mark
striatal patches (darkfield). B) CaBP immunoreactive labeling
of striatal matrix projection neurons (brightfield).

Corticostriatal inputs

We have examined the compartmental organization of cortico-
striatal systems in the rat (7,9) using Phaseolus vulgaris-leu-
coagglutinin (PHA-L) and autoradiographic axonal tract tracing
techniques (3,13), combined respectively with labeling of the
matrix with somatostatin-fiber immunoreactivity and labeling of
the patches with autoradiographic ligand binding of mu opiate
receptors. The prelimbic cortex, a cortical area on the medial
bank of the prefrontal cortex, projects throughout the striatum
but restricts its inputs to the patches. The cingulate cortex
also provides widespread striatal inputs but selectively innervates the matrix. Other cortical areas, such as motor and
sensory areas, provide striatal inputs relatively restricted in
area and distributed in a topographic manner in the matrix (7).
Studies in the monkey (16) and cat (36) provide similar views of
corticostriate compartmental organization.

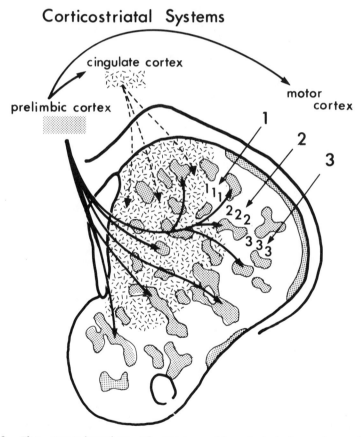

FIG. 2. The organization of some corticostriatal systems (7,9).

The topographic organization of corticostriatal projections is such that each striatal area receives inputs from cortical areas proximal to it. This is most evident in the projections of the motor and sensory cortical areas (29), but even these areas provide inputs to a striatal domain that is larger than to be expected if corticostriatal projections merely remapped the cortex in the striatum. Cortical areas with widespread cortical projections have widespread striatal projections, especially in the longitudinal axis (37,40), which results in extensive overlap of afferents from different cortical areas in any given striatal area. Our own studies suggest that the interactions of such widespread corticostriate projections are determined, in part, by the striatal patch-matrix organization. For instance, the prelimbic cortex, which projects to layer VI of most of the cerebral cortex and to most of the striatal patch system, projects to individual patches that are surrounded by matrix regions receiving inputs from cortical areas, such as the motor and cingulate cortices, with which the prelimbic cortex is itself interconnected (7,9).

Striatonigral Projection Systems

There is a rough topographic order in the striatonigral projections that maintains, in part, the relationship of striatal efferents in the mediolateral axis and inverts them in the dorsoventral axis (20,31,39). The inversion in this projection provides ventral striatal innervation of the substantia nigra pars compacta, the site of origin of the dopaminergic feedback system to the dorsal striatum (20,31). Recent studies in our laboratory have shown that as is the case of the corticostriatal system, striatonigral projections are divergent in nature and compartmentalized (9,11). Thus, while there is a rough topographic order, projections from restricted striatal regions are widespread in all axes of the substantia nigra, particularly longitudinally, providing extensive overlap of nigral afferents from regionally separated striatal areas.

Two distinct striatonigral systems arise from the patch and matrix compartments (9,11,12). The projections from the patches, even those from the dorsal patches, are directed to the pars compacta, whereas the projections of the matrix are directed to the pars reticulata. The dichotomy of patch and matrix striatonigral projections systems, originally identified with neuroanatomical tract tracing techniques, has been confirmed with the discovery of a biochemical marker that selectively labels the striatal matrix, and not the patch projection system. Calcium binding protein (CaBP) immunoreactivity is localized, in the striatum, in striatonigral projection neurons that are in the matrix while it is absent in the patches (12). CaBP immunoreactivity also labels the projections of matrix neurons and in the substantia nigra is localized in terminals in the pars reticulata. CaBP is absent in terminals in the pars compacta and in

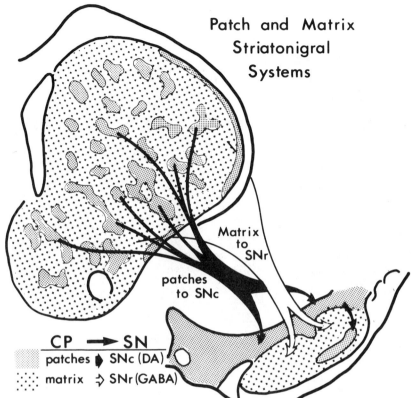

Patch and Matrix Striatonigral Systems

Matrix to SNr

patches to SNc

CP → SN
patches ▸ SNc (DA)
matrix ⇢ SNr (GABA)

FIG. 3. Diagram of separate patch and matrix striatonigral systems providing inputs, respectively, to the site of dopaminergic (DA) neurons in the substantia nigra pars compacta (SNc) and GABA containing neurons in the pars reticulata (SNr).

those areas of the pars reticulata where dopaminergic neurons are located (shaded area in ventrolateral SNr in Fig. 3). The pattern of CaBP immunoreactivity is in marked contrast to the distribution of substance P immunoreactivity. Substance P is localized in both patch and matrix projection systems (19,27) and in the substantia nigra labels afferents that overlap both the pars compacta and pars reticulata (12,25). Furthermore, retrograde tracing studies show that the labeled dendrites of striatonigral projection neurons are confined to the compartment in which their cell bodies are located (11). This is consistent with the report by Penny et al. (33) that intracellular filling of medium spiny striatal neurons, presumed projection neurons, have dendrites confined within one compartment or the other. Taken together with the compartmental organization of corticostriatal inputs this suggests that the patch and matrix compartments are segregated input-output pathways for cortical information processing by the striatum (9).

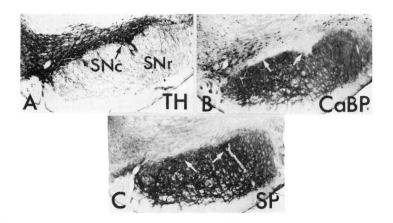

FIG. 4. Adjacent nigral sections to show relationship of TH (A),
CaBP (B) and substance P (C) immunoreactivity.

Striatal somatostatin interneurons

Somatostatin immunoreactivity labels a class of medium aspiny
striatal neurons that do not project outside the striatum and are
thus considered to be striatal interneurons (6,9,11,38). Although the majority of somatostatin immunoreactive neurons are
in the matrix (17) a substantial number of these extend dendrites
into the patches and there are a substantial number of somatostatin neurons that are themselves located in the patches (9,
11). Somatostatin fibers are distributed preferentially in the
matrix and even those patch neurons containing somatostatin
extend axons that ramify outside of the patches in the surrounding matrix (9,11). Thus, whereas corticostriatal input and
striatonigral output systems appear to maintain a segregation of
patch-matrix systems, some of the somatostatin interneurons may
provide a one way system linking the patches to the matrix.
Other striatal interneurons, such as the large cholinergic neurons (2), may also provide a linkage of patch and matrix.

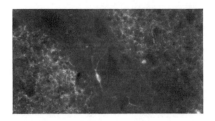

FIG. 5. Somatostatin immunoreactive neuron in a striatal patch
with fibers distributed to surrounding matrix areas.

Mesostriatal afferent systems

During development dopamine is first distributed in patches in the striatum and subsequently is distributed homogeneously in both patch and matrix compartments (32). We have examined the differential projections of subsets of midbrain dopaminergic and nondopaminergic neurons to the striatal patch and matrix compartments in the adult rat using axonal tracing techniques (10,14, 23). PHA-L injections into the substantia nigra label at least three morphologically distinct mesostriatal afferent fiber types. The two predominant fiber types labeled, types A and B differ primarily in size (type A: 0.1-0.3 μm and type B: 0.4-0.7 μ m), but are similar in ramifying into a plexiform pattern of fibers with boutons en passant that are only slightly larger than the diameter of the fibers themselves. The third fiber type, type C, is characterized by relatively large diameter fibers (0.7 μm), which ramify into distinct tree like arbors that terminate with large bulbous boutons (1.5 μm). Colocalization studies of tyrosine hydroxylase (TH) immunoreactivity in PHA-L labeled mesostriatal afferents show that fiber types A and B contain TH and are presumed to be dopaminergic whereas fiber type C does not contain TH and is presumed to be nondopaminergic (14). The morphological features of PHA-L labeled TH immunoreactive fibers are similar to those of TH immunoreactive striatal afferents identified at the electron microscopic level (1,35). The distribution of the different PHA-L labeled striatal afferent fiber types was compared in adjacent sections to the pattern of 3H-Naloxone binding to mark striatal patches. The ventral tegmental area (A10) provides dopaminergic fibers primarily to the matrix of the ventral striatum including the nucleus accumbens (see also ref. 23). Similarly, the retrorubral area (A8) provides dopaminergic fibers to the matrix and primarily to dorsal striatal regions. Dopaminergic inputs from the substantia nigra

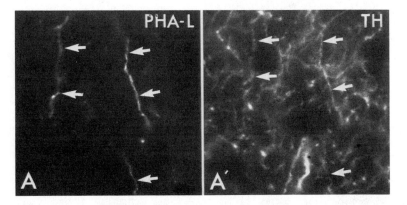

FIG. 6. (A) Transported PHA-L in nigrostriatal fiber type A that is colocalized with TH immunoreactivity (A') (14).

are distributed in both patch and matrix. Some nigral injections
label an input to both the patches and matrix while some, primarily those that label dopaminergic projections from neurons
in the pars reticulata , label inputs directed preferentially
to the patches. CaBP immunoreactivity, in addition to labeling
matrix projections to the pars reticulata, also labels midbrain
dopaminergic neurons that project to the striatal matrix (12).
The distribution of these neurons matches what might be expected
from the tracing studies. Thus, the majority of A10 and A8 dopaminergic neurons contain CaBP immunoreactivity while only subsets of pars compacta and a few pars reticulata dopaminergic
neurons also contain CaBP. Consequently, TH immunoreactive neurons that do not contain CaBP (TH+/CaBP-) appear to project to
the patches. In the pars compacta such neurons are interspersed
with neurons that project to the matrix. Nondopaminergic striatal afferents from both the VTA and substantia nigra are
distributed primarily in matrix areas.

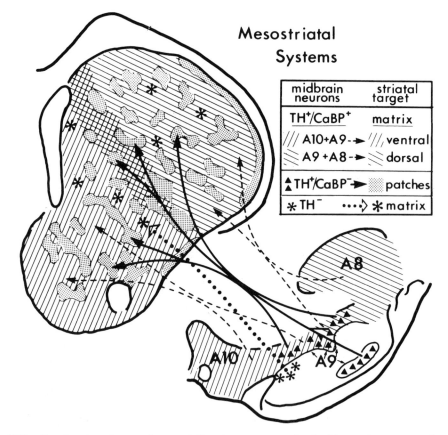

FIG. 7. Projections from midbrain areas, including the ventral
tegmental area (A10), substantia nigra (A9) and retrorubral area
(A8), to the striatum.

Discussion

The patch-matrix compartmental organization of the striatum provides parallel, segregated input-output pathways for processing cortical inputs through to the output nuclei of the basal ganglia, including the substantia nigra. The striatal matrix receives inputs from motor, somatosensory and cingulate cortical areas and projects to the location of GABAergic neurons in the substantia nigra pars reticulata, neurons that project to the thalamus, superior colliculus and midbrain tegmentum. Striatal patches receive inputs from the prelimbic cortex, a cortical area that receives direct inputs from limbic brain areas including the amygdala and hippocampus (28). Projections arising from the patches, even those in the dorsal striatum, selectively innervate dopaminergic neurons in the substantia nigra pars compacta, which are the source of the nigrostriatal feedback system. The compartmental organization of both corticostriatal input and striatonigral output systems suggests a segregation of input-output pathways, however, there are at least two types of systems that link the compartments. Somatostatin interneurons provide a potential substrate for interactions of patches with surrounding matrix regions locally. Additionally, nigrostriatal dopaminergic neurons, receiving striatal inputs principally from the patches, provide inputs to both the patch and matrix compartments.

Each subregion of the striatum, encompassing a domain that includes local patch and matrix areas, can be considered a local processing unit. These units are reiterated throughout the striatum, each with the common connectional features outlined above, although the specific connections vary from region to region. This organization of the striatum has several implications when considering the manner by which the striatum processes cortical inputs. First, the concept of regional specialization of the striatum is firmly grounded in the topographic organization of some its connections (21,26,31). Most notably the ventral striatum has been linked with limbic functions whereas the dorsal striatum is linked with sensorimotor (non-limbic) functions. However, the divergent and compartmental organization of certain corticostriate systems, for example those of the prelimbic cortex, suggests a more widely dispersed limbic influence throughout dorsal and ventral regions. In fact, although there is an underlying topography, studies point to the divergent nature of both corticostriatal (15,37,40) and striatonigral (11) systems that serve to provide for interaction of widely separated cortical inputs throughout the striatum and subsequently in the output targets of the basal ganglia by way of nigral inputs to the thalamus and superior colliculus. Although divergent in nature corticostriatal projections are not homogeneous such that each subregion of the striatum receives a different set of overlapping inputs from different cortical areas (37,40). Similarly striatonigral projections are divergent but not homogenous such that adjacent striatal matrix neurons may project to completely different loci in the substantia nigra while very distant striatal neurons may provide convergent inputs to the same nigral locus (11). This complex organization, with an underlying topography overlain with divergent/convergent connections, presumably accounts for reports of dissimilar physiologic response properties of adjacent neurons in the substantia nigra (24) and in thalamic and tectal targets of nigral inputs (5). As there is little direct interaction between distant striatal regions, it is the summation of the convergent outflow of the reiterated striatal patch-matrix subregions that presumably regulates the efferent output of individual nigral neurons. In this manner the basal ganglia are superbly organized to integrate all the diverse types of inputs from the cerebral cortex to affect behavior.

This paper is dedicated to the memory of Dr. Ed Evarts whose insights into brain function continue to provide inspiration for our work on the basal ganglia.

REFERENCES

1. Arluison, M., Dietl, M., and Thibault, J. (1984) Brain Res., 13: 269-285.
2. Bolam, J.P., Wainer, B.H., and Smith, A.D. (1984) Neuroscience, 12: 711-718.
3. Cowan, W.M., Gottlieb, D.L., Hendrickson, A.E., Price, J.L., and Woolsey, T.A. (1972) Brain Res., 37: 21-51.
4. Delong, M.R., Georgeopoulos, A.P., Crutcher, M.D., Mitchell, S.J. Richardson, R.T., and Alexander, G.E. (1984) In: Functions of the Basal Ganglia, edited by D. Evered and M. O'Connor, pp. 64-77, Pitman, London.
5. Deniau, J.M. and Chevalier, G. (1985) Brain Res., 334: 227-233.
6. DiFiglia, M. and Aronin, N. (1982) J. Neurosci., 2:1267-1274.
7. Donoghue,J.P. and Herkenham, M. (1983) Soc. Neurosci. Abstr., 9:11.
8. Evarts,E.V. (1984) In: Functions of the Basal Ganglia, edited by D. Evered and M. O'Connor, pp.1-2, Pitman, London.
9. Gerfen, C.R. (1984) Nature, 311:461-464.
10. Gerfen, C.R. (1984) Soc. Neurosci. Abstr., 10:9.
11. Gerfen, C.R. (1985) J. Comp. Neurol., 236:454-476.
12. Gerfen, C.R., Baimbridge, K.G., and Miller, J.J. (1985) Proc. Natl. Acad. Sci. (USA), in press.
13. Gerfen, C.R. and Sawchenko, P.E. (1984) Brain Res., 290: 219-238.
14. Gerfen, C.R. and Sawchenko, P.E. (1985) Brain Res., 343:144-150.
15. Goldman, P.S. and Nauta, W.J.H. (1977) J. Comp. Neurol., 171-369-386.

16. Goldman-Rakic, P.S. (1982) J. Comp. Neurol., 205: 398-413.
17. Graybiel, A.M., Ragsdale, C.W., Yoneoka, E.S., and Elde, R.H. (1981) Neuroscience, 6: 377-397.
18. Graybiel, A.M. and Ragsdale, C.W. (1978) Proc. Natl. Acad. Sci. (USA), 75: 5723-5726.
19. Graybiel, A.M. and Chesselet, M.F. (1984) Proc. Natl. Acad. Sci. (USA), 81: 7980-7984.
20. Grofova, I. (1979) In: The Neostriatum, edited by I. Divac and R.G.E. Oberg, pp. 37-51, Pergamon Press, Oxford.
21. Heimer, L. and Wilson, R.D. (1975) In: Golgi Centennial Symposium, edited by M. Santini, pp. 177-193, Raven Press, New York.
22. Herkenham, M. and Pert, C.B. (1981) Nature, 291: 415-418.
23. Herkenham, M., Moon-Edley, S., and Stuart, J. (1984) Neuroscience, 11: 561-593.
24. Hikosaka, H. and Wurtz, R.H. (1983) J. Neurophysiol. 49: 1268-1284.
25. Inagaki, S. and Parent, A. (1984) Brain Res. Bull. 13: 319-329.
26. Kelley, A.E., Domesick, V.B. and Nauta, W.J.H. (1982) Neuroscience 7: 615-630.
27. Kohno, J., Shiosaka, S., Shinoda, K., Inagaki, S., and Tohyama, M. (1984) Brain Res. 308: 308-317.
28. Krettek, J.E. and Price, J.L. (1978) J. Comp. Neurol. 178: 255-280.
29. Kunzle, H. (1975) Brain Res. 88: 195-209.
30. Liles, S.L. (1978) Fed. Proc. Abstr. 37: 396.
31. Nauta, W.J.H., Smith, G.P., Faull, R.L.M., and Domesci, V.B. (1978) Neuroscience, 3: 385-401.
32. Olson, L., Seiger, A., and Fuxe, K., (1972) Brain Res. 44: 283-288.
33. Penney, G.R., Wilson, C.J., and Kitai, S.T. (1984) Soc. Neurosci. Abstr. 10: 514.
34. Pert, C.B., Kuhar, M. J., and Synder, S.H. (1976) Proc. Natl. Acad. Sci. (USA) 73: 3729-3733.
35. Pickel, V.M., Beckley, S.C., Joh, T.J., and Reis, D.J. (1981) Brain Res, 225: 373-385.
36. Ragsdale, C.W., and Graybiel, A.M. (1981) Brain Res. 208: 259-266.
37. Selemon, L.D. and Goldman-Rakic, P.S. (1985) Neuroscience, 5: 776-794.
38. Takagi, H., Somogyi, P., Somagyi, J., and Smith, A.D. (1983) J. Comp. Neurol., 214: 1-16.
39. Tulloch, I.F., Arbuthnott, G.W., and Wright, A.K. (1978) J. Anat. 127: 425-441.
40. Yeterian, E.H. and Van Hoesen, G.W. (1978) Brain Res. 139: 43-63.

*Neurotransmitter Interactions in the Basal
Ganglia,* edited by M. Sandler et al.
Raven Press, New York © 1987.

MORPHOMETRICAL AND MICRODENSITOMETRICAL STUDIES ON THE MOSAIC
ORGANIZATION OF THE STRIATUM. FOCUS ON NEUROPEPTIDE/DOPAMINE
TRANSMITTER INTERACTIONS AT THE PRE- AND POSTSYNAPTIC LEVEL

KJELL FUXE, [1]LUIGI F. AGNATI, [1]MICHELE ZOLI, ANDERS HÄRFSTRAND,
[2]SVEN-OVE ÖGREN, [1]EMILIO MERLO PICH, [1]ISABELLA ZINI AND [3]MENEK
GOLDSTEIN

Dept. of Histology, Karolinska Institutet, Stockholm, Sweden.
Dept. of Human Physiology Univ. of Modena, Modena, Italy[1].
ASTRA Pharmaceuticals, Södertälje, Sweden[2] and Dept. of
Psychiatry, New York Univ. Medical Center, New York, USA[3].

In 1971 in an analysis of the postnatal neostriatum by means
of catecholamine (CA) fluorescence histochemistry it became
clear that the nigrostriatal dopamine (DA) neurons may form
different types of nerve terminal systems in the neostriatum
(7). Thus, in addition to the well known homogeneous plexus of
DA terminals innervating the neostriatum brightly fluorescent
islands of densely packed DA nerve terminals were demonstrated
in the dorsal striatum (DA islands or striosomes), (see also
17). Subsequent histochemical and pharmacological studies gave
further evidence for this hypothesis (9, 10, 11, 20, 23). These
early studies also presented the first indication for the
existence of a mosaic organization of the neostriatum (see also
Gerfen, this symposium) superimposed on diffuse networks (the
even "matrix").

In the present article we will summarize our recent work on
the organization of the nigrostriatal DA neurons at the pre-
and postsynaptic level and their interactions with neuropeptides such as neurotensin, enkephalines and neuropeptide Y
(NPY). The role of neuropeptides in the intra- and intersynaptic regulation of DA receptors will be especially discussed.

PRE- AND POSTSYNAPTIC FEATURES OF STRIATAL DA SYNAPSES IN
RELATION TO THE MOSAIC ORGANIZATION OF THE STRIATUM.

In fig. 1 the brightly fluorescent DA islands are shown in
the dorsomedial striatum of the 7 day old male rat. Upon the
subsequent postnatal development of the striatal DA innervation
these islands become masked, since also the diffusely distributed (matrix) DA nerve terminal networks become strongly
fluorescent as revealed by the CA fluorescence method of Falck
and Hillarp. However, in the adult animal they can easily be
demonstrated by means of tyrosine hydroxylase (TH) immunocytochemistry (15). Thus, these islands are characterized by
high amounts of TH immunoreactivity, which makes it possible to
observe TH immunoreactive (IR) islands and striae, since the

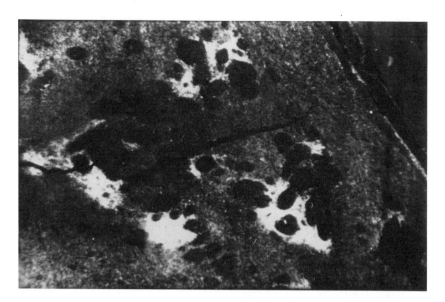

Fig. 1   Strongly fluorescent CA nerve terminal islands are
observed in the striatum of the 7 day old male rat as demonstrated by CA fluorescence histochemistry.   The medial part of
the nucleus caudatus is shown close to the lateral ventricle
(V).   Dorsal is upwards. The weakly fluorescent CA terminals
located in the surrounding matrix in the striatum represent the
diffuse type of DA nerve terminals which at this stage of
development is not fully developed. x120.

matrix DA nerve terminals contain less TH immunoreactivity. In
1982 it became possible for the first time to objectively
describe the DA island by analyzing the TH IR striatal terminals by means of computer-assisted microdensitometry and
morphometry (1). In this analysis it could be demonstrated that
the TH IR islands and striae, are characterized by densely
packed DA nerve terminals having high amounts of TH immunoreactivity and DA (see fig. 2). The nerve cells of these DA
islands also contain high amounts of DA and CAMP regulated
phosphoprotein-32 (DARPP-32, Fuxe, Agnati, Härfstrand, Quimet,
Hemmings, Walaas, Goldstein and Greengard, to be published). A
rostrocaudal analysis of the TH IR nerve terminals in the
neostriatum has also been performed with regard to their
relative optical density (see fig. 3). It is shown that the DA
nerve terminals of the islands at all rostrocaudal levels show
a higher degree of TH immunoreactivity than that found in the
diffusely distributed TH IR terminals. DA nerve terminals of
the islands or striosomes have previously also been shown to
have a lower DA utilization than the matrix DA nerve terminals
(fig. 2; 10).
    By means of quantitative receptor autoradiography we have
also analyzed using ^{3}H-spiperone (D2 antagonist) and ^{3}H-SCH

SCHEME OF DA INNERVATION OF STRIATUM

	TH-IR	DA CONTENT	DA TURNOVER	DARPP IR
STRIAE ISLANDIC TYPE	+ +	+ +	Low	+ +
DIFFUSE TYPE	+	+	High	+

Fig. 2   Schematical illustration of the neurochemical properties of the striatal DA nerve terminals of the islands and
of the matrix (diffuse type).

**ROSTRO-CAUDAL ANALYSIS OF TH-POSITIVE TERMINALS
IN STRIATUM**

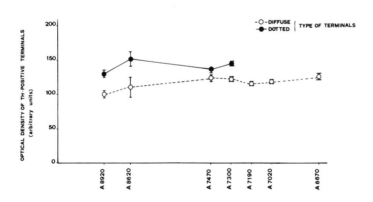

Fig. 3   Rostrocaudal analysis of TH immunoreactivity in the
diffuse and dotted type of DA nerve terminals in the striatum.
By microdensitometrical measurements optical density in the TH
IR nerve terminals has been determined (expressed in arbitrary
units), giving an evaluation of the relative TH immunoreactivity. Means + s.e.m. are shown at various rostrocaudal levels
(König and Klippel Atlas). n = 3. For details on the methodology, see 3.

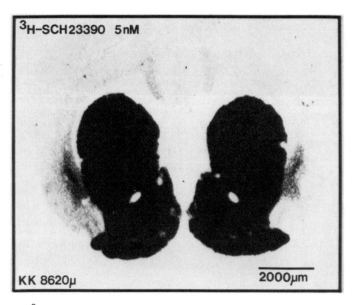

Fig. 4   ^{3}H-SCH23390 receptor autoradiogram of an adult male rat. The strong diffuse labelling of the neostriatum, nucleus accumbens and tuberculum olfactorium is shown. The autoradiogram in these areas has been over exposed in order to more clearly demonstrate the labelling in the claustrum.

23390 (D1 antagonist) as radioligands, if the DA islands or striosomes have a postsynaptic correlate. However, as seen in figs. 4 and 5 the D1 receptors and D2 receptors in the neostriatum, tuberculum olfactorium and nucleus accumbens are not distributed in a patchy fashion. The binding results in a relatively diffuse labelling of the entire dorsal and ventral striatum. Furthermore, ^{3}H-SCH 23390 is shown to substantially label the claustrum indicating that this region is rich in D1 receptors. As seen in fig. 5, however, there is no homogeneous distribution of the D2 receptors which is true also for the D1 receptors. Thus, a substantially higher degree of specific binding of ^{3}H-spiperone is found in the lateral part compared with the medial part at all rostrocaudal levels analyzed. The highest labelling is found in the dorsolateral part of the neostriatum at all rostrocaudal levels analyzed (3). The D1 receptors appear to have a similar type of distribution as illustrated in fig. 4, but the quantitative analysis has not yet been completed (see also Scatton, this symposium).
 Automatic image analysis has also been used to study the distribution of TH and enkephalin (ENK) IR nerve cell bodies and terminals and the overlap among TH-IR and ENK-IR islands (see Table 1). To this aim the coronal view of the striatum has been subdivided into a marginal zone (a strip 500 μm wide

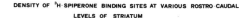

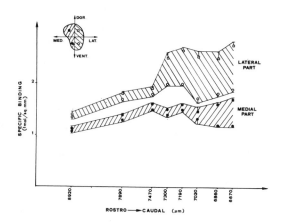

Fig. 5   Studies on the distribution of ^{3}H-spiperone labelled
DA receptors in the nucleus caudatus putamen at various rostrocaudal levels (König and Klippel Atlas). The results obtained
are based on an analysis of ^{3}H-spiperone receptor autoradiograms obtained from coronal sections of the diencephalon at
various rostrocaudal levels. For details on the methodology see
3. The concentration of ^{3}H-spiperone was 2 nM. Specific binding
has been measured in the 4 quadrants shown in the fig., expressed in fmol/sq.mm. Means ± s.e.m. are shown. n = 4.

around the striatal border) and a central zone (the rest of the
striatum). Furthermore the distribution of NPY IR cell bodies
in the neostriatum has been analyzed. It has not been possible
to demonstrate a significant gradient of increasing densities
of ENK IR nerve cell bodies as the sampling field (square 150
or 255 μm by side) moves medially to laterally in the neostriatum or dorsally to ventrally. On the contrary a significant gradient could be demonstrated for the TH-IR nerve terminals. Thus, TH-IR tends to decrease according to a dorsoventral axis.

We have also discovered a substantial (about 20%) overlap
between the DA nerve terminal striae and the ENK IR striae in
the striatum (see Table 1, analysis at marginal zone level).
However, interestingly the ENK IR nerve terminal islands within
the central part of the neostriatum show only a minor relationship to the striatal DA islands. These results clearly indicate
that there exist heterogeneities in the neurochemistry of the
striatal islands.

TABLE 1

This analysis has been carried out by means of computer-assisted morphometry and microdensitometry. To visualize islands an interactive discrimination procedure followed by a close function to assess boundaries of the islands has been performed. It should be pointed out that the vibratom section thickness was 35 μm. Thus, the overlap values are an underestimation due to the spatial displacement of the neuronal structures. For this type of problem a correlation factor can be used as demonstrated by Agnati et al. (3). Marginal zone = a 500 μm wide zone making up the periphery of striatum on the medial, dorsal and lateral side. Central zone = the remaining part of the striatum.

Striatal immunoreactivity (IR)	Gradients		Entity of islandic-IR (% of total IR)		Overlap of IR-islands (% of TH-IR islands)	
	mediolateral	dorsoventral	marginal zone	central zone	marginal zone	central zone
TH-IR	NO	YES (decreasing)	30%	5%	——	——
ENK-IR	NO	NO	18%	10%	20%	5%

It follows, also, that the ENK and the TH IR islands predominantly interact with non dopaminergic and non-enkephalinergic terminal systems. Of substantial interest is the observation that ENK IR cell bodies exist both inside and outside the ENK IR islands. The islands and the striosomes may represent important integrative units in the striatum, the neurochemical characteristics of which may vary depending upon their topographical localization and their input-output projections. The available evidence suggests that the islands or striosomes predominantly send axons to the substantia nigra (see Gerfen this symposium). In the case of the ENK islands there may also exist a postsynaptic correlate, since a patchy labelling is observed in the striatum (3) using ^{3}H-etorphine and ^{3}H-D-ALA^2-D-LEU^5-Enkephalin as radioligands for mμ and delta receptors, respectively. However, it remains to be shown that there exists an overlap between the ENK IR nerve terminal islands and the patches of receptors formed in the receptor autoradiograms. It may be suggested that the mosaic organization of the striatum may be analogous to the columnar organization of the cerebral cortex.

In figs. 6 and 7 a scatter diagram and a density map are shown of the distribution of NPY IR nerve cell bodies in the entire striatum as shown in a coronal section of the rat brain at the König and Klippel level A 8380. These maps were obtained

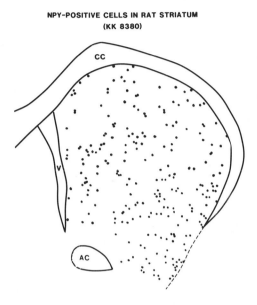

NPY-POSITIVE CELLS IN RAT STRIATUM
(KK 8380)

Fig. 6   A scatter diagram is shown demonstrating the distribution of NPY IR nerve cells in the rat striatum at König and
Klippel level A 8380. The NPY IR cells were demonstrated by the
indirect immunoperoxidase procedure. V = lateral ventricle; CC
= corpus callosum; AC = anterior limb of the anterior commi-
sure. Each point represents a NPY IR nerve cell body.

by analysis of sections stained for NPY-like immunoreactivity
(6). As seen the NPY-like IR nerve cell bodies appear to be
relatively evenly distributed all over the striatum and the
density is low compared with e. g. the ENK IR nerve cell
bodies. Thus, there exists a low density of NPY IR profiles all
over the striatum. The NPY IR cell bodies do not form clusters
but may be a neuronal element in most - if not all - of the
various striosomes located in the striatal matrix. Thus, the
NPY IR neurons of the striatum may have the similar role as the
VIP IR neurons of the microcolumns of the cerebral cortex.
Within the cerebral cortex the vasoactive intestinal polypeptide (VIP) IR neurons appear to represent 1% of the total
nerve cell population (18).
    The existence of DA islands with precise interactions with
other types of transmitter identified nerve terminals contrasts
with the presence of apparently diffusely distributed dopaminergic networks all over the striatum. Thus, the information

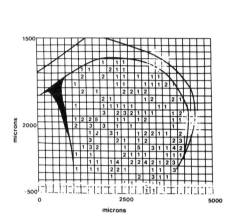

NPY-POSITIVE CELLS IN STRIATUM (KK8380)

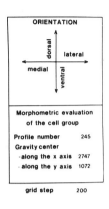

ORIENTATION

dorsal   lateral

medial

ventral

Morphometric evaluation
of the cell group

Profile number	245
Gravity center	
- along the x axis	2747
- along the y axis	1072
grid step	200

Fig. 7   A density map is shown of the distribution of NPY IR
nerve cells in the striatum. The density map was obtained by
analysis of the scatter diagram illustrated in fig. 6. The
unitary square used in this density map has a side of 200 μm.

handling in the basal ganglia and probably in the CNS as a
whole may depend upon at least two different types of transmission (4, 14). The various mosaics in the striatum may mainly
represent the neuron linked electrochemical transmission, which
depends upon the precise wiring of the network (wiring of
transmission) (fig. 8). Instead the diffuse networks of DA
terminals of the striatum may mainly operate via humoral (open)
electrochemical transmission. Thus, in this case the transmitter and cotransmitters reach a certain volume of striatal
tissue, in which the receptors for their transmitter and
peptide cotransmitters and their fragments are activated. In
this way the neuronal network is liberated from the constraints
of the neuroanatomical wiring of the network (see fig. 8). This
type of transmission has a low safety and low speed but shows
a high degree of divergency and of plasticity. An holistic
elaboration and a long term action is obtained.

It must also be emphasized that the striatal nerve cells both
within the striatal mosaic and in the striatal matrix probably
are under important endocrine control in view of our recent
observations showing the existence of glucocorticoid receptor
immunoreactivity in the majority of the striatal nerve cell
bodies (13). Thus, the metabolic state as well as the responsi-
vity of the cells to neuronal signals both via the "wiring of
transmission" and the "volume of transmission" is regulated by

KIND OF TRANSMISSION	SPEED OF TRANSMISSION	DEGREE OF DIVERGENCE	SEGREGATION ("safety" of the transmission)	PLASTICITY	PREFERENTIAL INFORMATION PROCESSING
"wiring" neuron linked electro-chemical transmission	high	low to moderate	high	low	elementary elaboration short term action
"volume of transmission" humoral ("open") electro-chemical transmission	low	high to very high	low	high	holistic elaboration long term action

Fig. 8   Characterization of two different types of electro-chemical transmission in the central nervous system: the wiring of transmission and the volume of transmission.

the endocrine system, probably mainly via the glucocorticoid hormones.

INDICATIONS FOR A POSSIBLE UNIQUE RECEPTOR MECHANISM IN THE DA MOSAIC UNIT IN THE STRIATUM

In previous work (8, 9) it was demonstrated that the ergolene derivative MPME (PTR17402; 5R,8R-8 - (4-p-methoxyphenyl-1-piper-azinylmethyl)-6-methylergolene) reduces DA utilization exclus-ively within the striosomes of the striatum, and in the dotted DA-CCK costoring terminals of the nucleus accumbens and the olfactory tubercle. These results indicate the existence of DA receptors in the islands, which can be differentially activated by a dopaminergic agonist such as MPME. In these papers it was also shown that MPME activates striatal adenylate cyclase, indicating that MPME at least can activate the D1 type of DA receptor (8, 9). In view of these interesting properties of this ergolene derivative we have recently studied the be-havioural properties of MPME (24). It was found that the drug induced a characteristic behavioural syndrome consisting of increased locomotion, head bobbing and sniffing activity without oral stereotypies or increased rearing. Unselective DA receptor antagonists but not selective D2 receptor antagonists such as remoxipride and sulpiride could significantly block the locomotion and head bobbing behaviour induced by MPME. A blockade of the locomotor syndrome induced by MPME has also recently been observed after pretreatment with the D1 anta-

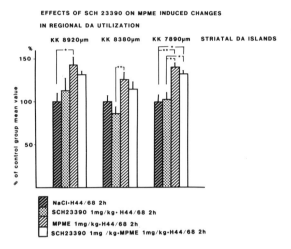

EFFECTS OF SCH 23390 ON MPME INDUCED CHANGES
IN REGIONAL DA UTILIZATION

Fig. 9   Effects of a Dl receptor antagonist SCH 23390 on MPME induced changes in DA utilization in DA striatal islands at various rostrocaudal levels. The DA utilization was evaluated by the use of the TH inhibitor α—methyl-tyrosine-methylester (H44/68), which was administered 2 h before killing in a dose of 250 mg/kg i.p. MPME in a dose of 1 mg/kg, given i.p. immediately after the injection of H44/68, induces a significant reduction of DA utilization in all the striatal islands analyzed. This action was not significantly counteracted by the Dl receptor antagonist. Means $\pm$ s.e.m. n = 6. In the statistical analysis Wilcoxon test, comparing all possible pairs of treatments, was used. * = $p<0.05$; ** = $p<0.01$. All values are expressed in % of the control group mean value treated with the H44/68 alone. The respective basal values expressed in nmol/g of w.w. of tissue are as follows: 190, 175 and 186 at König and Klippel levels 8920, 8390 and 7890 μm respectively.

gonist SCH 23390. These results indicated that Dl receptor activation in the forebrain, perhaps mainly linked to some types of DA systems, can produce behavioural actions, which differ from those produced by activation of D2 receptors in the forebrain (24). Thus, a "Dl syndrome" is introduced.

As seen in fig. 9 we have now continued the analysis of the properties of this interesting ergolene derivative. As seen the reduction of DA utilization produced by MPME in the striosomes at various rostrocaudal levels of the neostriatum cannot be antagonized by simultaneous treatment with a high dose of the Dl receptor antagonist SCH 23390. By itself the Dl receptor antagonist does not change the DA utilization as evaluated in

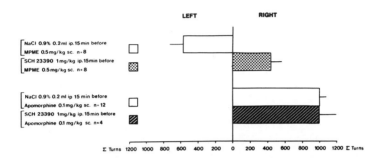

Fig. 10 Studies on rotational behaviour after administration of the dopaminergic ergot drug MPME or apomorphine in rats with nigral 6-hydroxydopamine induced lesions on the left side. Means + s.e.m. are shown. The treatment schedules are shown. The columns represent the total number of turns made towards the right or the left side. Turns towards the right side indicate activation of supersensitive DA receptors probably of the D2 type on the lesioned side. In contrast the turning behaviour induced by MPME towards the left side (ipsilateral rotational behaviour) may be induced via activation of supersensitive D1 receptors having an opposite functional action to that of the D2 receptors.

the TH inhibition model. In these experiments α-methyl-tyrosine-methylester (α-MT) was given immediately before the administration of the drugs in a dose of 250 mg/kg (i.p., 2 hours before killing). In previous work (9) it was shown that haloperidol could counteract the reduction of DA utilization by MPME in the striosomes. Thus, these results indicate that the behavioural syndrome induced by MPME is produced via a D1 receptor, while the selective reduction of DA utilization in the striosomes may be related to activation of a special type of D2 autoreceptor present on the DA terminals of the DA islands. In line with this interpretation our recent results show that PTR17402 has a high affinity for the striatal ^{3}H-spiperone binding sites, which represent D2 receptors (IC 50 19.3 nM). These results suggest that MPME may interact with D2 receptors as a partial agonist.

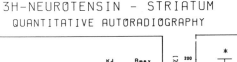

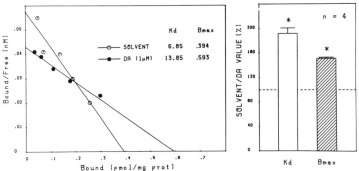

Fig. 11 Scatchard plots are shown to illustrate the effect of DA (1 μM) on ³H-Neurotensin binding in striatum using quantitative receptor autoradiography. The K_D values are given in nM and the B_{max} values in pmol/mg protein. In the right part the effects of DA of the ³H-neurotensin binding characteristics are summarized. Means ± s.e.m. out of 4 rats. Students paired t-test was used in the statistical analysis. * = p<0.05.

Taken together it therefore seems possible that the unique behavioural syndrome induced by MPME may be related to its ability to activate postsynaptic striatal D1 receptors at the same time as it may act as a partial D2 receptor agonist. Furthermore, its ability to preferentially reduce DA utilization in the islands may be caused by a preferential DA agonistic activity at presynaptic D2 receptors of the islandic DA nerve terminals. It is also possible that the preferential reduction of DA utilization in the islands can be related to a higher presynaptic receptor reserve in these DA terminals compared with the DA terminals of the matrix (16).

It is of special interest that MPME induces its characteristic D1 behavioural syndrome by being a D1 agonist and a partial D2 receptor agonist. In fact, a recent study has reported that a D1 receptor agonist SKF38393 can greatly enhance the ability of a low dose of a D2 receptor antagonist to induce abnormal perioral movements in rats (22). It has also been demonstrated that the D1 receptor antagonist SCH 23390 blocks DA induced CAMP formation in striatal homogenates, an action, which is counteracted by a D2 receptor antagonist (21). Interactive effects of D1 and D2 DA receptor blockade have also been demonstrated in vitro and in vivo by Salama and Saller (19).

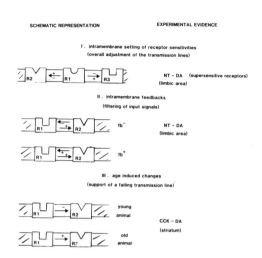

Fig. 12 Schematic illustration of possible functional roles of receptor-receptor interactions in information processing at the membrane level based on experimental evidence obtained in a series of paper summarized in 2, 12.

Recently we have also been able to obtain evidence for functional interactions between D1 and D2 receptors (Ögren, Holm and Fuxe, unpublished data). Thus, D2 receptor antagonists such as sulpiride and ethyclopride can in a dose dependent manner block apomorphine induced hypothermia. In contrast, SCH 23390 in various doses significantly enhances the apomorphine induced hypothermia, giving clear evidence for an opposing role of D1 and D2 receptors in the regulation of body temperature. In line with these results MPME produces ipsilateral and apomorphine contralateral rotational behaviour in rats with unilateral 60H-DA induced nigral lesions, giving evidence for opposite functional roles of striatal D1 and D2 receptors (fig. 10). After D1 receptor blockade the MPME induced ipsilateral rotational behavior is transferred into a contralateral rotational behaviour, probably controlled by supersensitive D2 receptors, which are activated by the partial agonistic properties of MPME at D2 receptors.

INTRA- AND INTERSYNAPTIC REGULATION OF STRIATAL DA RECEPTORS

Biochemical studies at a postsynaptic level have given evidence for the existence of a number of interactions between receptors in membrane preparations of the basal ganglia (2, 12). Thus, glutamate, cholecystokinin peptides and neurotensin can all regulate the binding characteristics of the striatal DA receptor. Interactions between neurotensin and DA receptors in the dorsal and ventral striatum have been shown to be bidirectional and been demonstrated also by means of quantitative autoradiography using ^{3}H-neurotensin as a radioligand and DA (1 µM) as a modulator (see fig. 11) (5). It is shown that DA can produce a significant and substantial increase in both the K_D-value and the B_{max} value of the ^{3}H-neurotensin binding sites in the striatum. It has been demonstrated that neurotensin (1-10 nM) reduces the affinity of the DA agonist binding sites in membrane preparations from the dorsal and ventral striatum (12). Thus, it seems possible that activation of DA receptors can lead to an increase in the neurotensin receptor mechanism, which in turn reduces the affinity of the DA agonist sites, in this way reducing DA transmission. These results therefore indicate that one role of receptor-receptor interaction may be to make possible intramembrane negative feedback loops, in this case controlling the sensitivity of the DA receptors (see fig. 12). In this way a filtering mechanism of input signals is obtained at the membrane level. Another role of interactions between receptors in the membrane may be an intramembrane setting of receptor sensitivities leading to an overall adjustment of the transmission lines (4) (fig. 12). Changes in the receptor-receptor interactions have also been noticed in relation to aging in studies on cholecystokinin-DA receptor interactions. Thus, in old age cholecystokinin peptides (CCK8) increases DA antagonist binding instead of reducing it as in the young animal. This altered modulation may be the result of a mechanism activated to support the failing DA transmission line in the old animal (4, 12).

In conclusion, the present results provide evidence for neurochemical heterogeneities in the mosaic organization of the striatum, as well as for a unique DA receptor mechanism in the stratal DA islands. The DA ergoline MPME is shown to induce a D1 locomotor syndrome. The evidence for an intersynaptic and intrasynaptic regulation of DA receptors via receptor-receptor interactions is summarized.

ACKNOWLEDGEMENTS

This work has been supported by a grant from the American Parkinson Foundation and by a CNR-international grant. For excellent technical assistance we are grateful to Barbro Tinner, Birgitta Nyberg, Ulla Britt Finnman, Kerstin Lundberg and Lars Rosén. For excellent secretarial assistance we are grateful to Anne Edgren and Rose Marie Gustafsson.

REFERENCES

1. Agnati, L.F., Fuxe, K., Zini, I., Calza, L., Benfenati, F., Zoli, M., Hökfelt, T., and Goldstein, M. (1982): Neurosci. Lett., 32:253-258.
2. Agnati, L.F., Fuxe, K., Benfenati, F., Battistini, N., Zini, I., Camurri, M., and Hökfelt, T. (1984): Neurology and Neurobiology, edited by E. Usdin, A. Carlsson, A. Dahlström, and J. Engel. Vol. 8B, pp. 191-198. Alan R. Liss Inc., New York.
3. Agnati, L.F., Fuxe, K., Benfenati, F., Zini, I., Zoli, M., Fabbri, L., and Härfstrand, A. (1984): Acta Physiol. Scand., 532 (Suppl.):5-36.
4. Agnati, L.F., Fuxe, K., Zoli, M., Merlo Pich, E., Benfenati, F., Zini, I., and Goldstein, M. (1985): Progress in Brain Res., (in press).
5. Benfenati, F., Agnati, L.F., and Fuxe, K. (1985): Acta Physiol. Scand., (in press).
6. Everitt, B.J., Hökfelt, T., Terenius, L., Tatemoto, K., Mutt, V., and Goldstein, M. (1984): Neuroscience Vol. 11, 2:443-462.
7. Fuxe, K., Hökfelt, T., and Ungerstedt, U. (1971): In: Monoamines Noyaux Gris Centraux et Syndrome de Parkinson, edited by J. Ajuriaguerra and G. Gauthier, pp. 23-60. Georg and S.A. Cie, Geneva.
8. Fuxe, K., Fredholm, B., Agnati, L.F., Ögren, S.-O., Everitt, B.J., Jonsson, G., and Gustafsson, J.-Å. (1978): Pharmacology 16:99-134.
9. Fuxe, K., Fredholm, B.P., Agnati, L.F., and Corrodi, H. (1978): Brain Res., 146:295-311.
10. Fuxe, K., Andersson, K., Schwarcz, R., Agnati, L.F., Perez de la Mora, M., Hökfelt, T., Goldstein, M., Ferland, L., Possani, I., and Tapia, R. (1979): In: Advances in Neurology, Vol. 24, edited by L.J. Piorier, T.L. Sourkes and P.J. Bédard, pp. 199-214. Raven Press, New York.
11. Fuxe, K., Agnati, L.F., Ögren, S.-O., Köhler, C., Calza, L., Benfenati, F., Goldstein, M., Andersson, K., and Eneroth, P. (1983): In: Symposium on Dopamine Receptor Agonists, edited by A. Carlsson and J.L.G. Nilsson, pp. 60-79. Swedish Pharmaceutical Press, Stockholm.
12. Fuxe, K. and Agnati, L.F. (1985): Med. Res. Rev., Vol. 5, 4:441-482.
13. Fuxe, K., Wikström, A.-C., Okret, S., Agnati, L.F., Härfstrand, A., Yu, Z.-Y., Granholm, L., Zoli, M., Vale, W., and Gustafsson, J.-Å. (1985): Endocrinology, Vol. 117, No. 5:1-11.
14. Fuxe, K., Agnati, L.F., Härfstrand, A., Janson, A.M., Neumeyer, A., Andersson, K., Ruggeri, M., Zoli, M., and Goldstein, M. (1985): Progress in Brain Res., (in press).
15. Fuxe, K., Agnati, L.F., Härfstrand, A., Ögren, S.-O., and

Goldstein, M. (1986): In: Recent Development in Parkinson's Disease, edited by S. Fahn, D. Marsden, P. Teychenne and P. Jenner, (in press). Raven Press, New York.

16. Goldstein, M., Kusano, N., Adler, C.,, and Meller, E. (1985): Progress in Brain Res., (in press).

17. Graybiel, A.M., Pickel, V.M., Joh, T.H., Reis, D.J., and Ragsdale, C.W. (1981): Proc. Natl. Acad. Sci., 78:5871-5875.

18. Morrison, J.H., and Bloom, F.E. (1985): In: Quantitative Neuroanatomy in Transmitter Research, edited by L.F. Agnati and K. Fuxe, (in press). MacMillan Press, London.

19. Saller, C.F. and Salama, A.I. (1985): Eur. J. Pharmacol., 109:297-300.

20. Olson, L., Seiger, Å., and Fuxe, K. (1972): Brain Res., 44:283-288.

21. Onali, P., Olianas, M.C., and Gessa, G.L. (1984): Eur. J. Pharmacol., 99:127-128.

22. Rosengarten, H., Schweitzer, J.W., and Friedhoff, A.J. (1983): Life Sci., 33:2479-2482.

23. Tennyson, V.M., Barrett, R.E., Cohen, G., Coté, L., Heikkila, R., and Mytilineou, C. (1972): Brain Res., 46:251-285.

24. Ögren, S.-O., Fuxe, K., Ängeby, K., and Köhler, C. (1985): Eur. J. Pharmacol., 106:79-89.

Neurotransmitter Interactions in the Basal Ganglia, edited by M. Sandler et al.
Raven Press, New York © 1987.

POSSIBLE SITES OF TRANSMITTER
INTERACTION IN THE NEOSTRIATUM: AN ANATOMICAL APPROACH

J.P.Bolam and P.N.Izzo

MRC Anatomical Neuropharmacology Unit,
Department of Pharmacology, South Parks Road, Oxford, OX1 3QT,
U.K.

The complexity of the neostriatum, among all regions of the basal ganglia, is exemplified by the rich diversity of neurotransmitters or neurotransmitter-markers that have been detected either within striatal neurons or within afferents of the striatum. In the region of 40 putative neurotransmitters or neuromodulators have been identified by a variety of techniques. (See reviews 20, 29). The figure is somewhat lower for the better established putative transmitters. There is strong evidence for populations of striatal neurons containing gamma aminobutyric acid (GABA), acetylcholine, substance P, somatostatin and an opiate peptide while afferents of the striatum include those containing glutamate (from the cortex), dopamine (from the substantia nigra) and 5-hydroxytryptamine (from the raphe). Taking this conservative estimate of the number of transmitters in the striatum, one can estimate the number of theoretical transmitter interactions ; this will be the number of transmitters squared. Thus with eight transmitters one can envisage that there are 64 possible sites of interaction (including autoactions). However this number is an under estimate because 1) there are probably many more than eight transmitters in the striatum and 2) this estimate only takes into account _direct_ effects of one transmitter upon another. In reality one transmitter may interact with another indirectly via disynaptic and multisynaptic routes and interactions may occur between two or more transmitters on the postsynaptic structures.

One way to study possible transmitter interactions and possible _sites_ of transmitter interactions is to establish circuit diagrams in which the morphology of individual neurons is directly correlated with its chemistry and the origin, chemistry and pattern of afferent synapses. By knowing the transmitter contained within a neuron, where this neuron makes synaptic contact and the transmitters and pattern of afferent synapses, not only can possible sites of transmitter interaction be identified but also possible sites of drug action may be obtained.

Of the nine morphologically distinct kinds of striatal neurons, (11) only five have been analysed by these methods to a greater or lesser extent. These include: 1) medium-size densely spiny neurons, 2) cholinergic interneurons, 3) GABA-synthesizing interneurons, 4) somatostatin-containing neurons and 5) a large pallidal-like neuron that projects to the substantia nigra. This paper will be confined to the first two classes, the medium-size densely spiny neurons and the cholinergic interneuron.

MEDIUM-SIZE DENSELY SPINY NEURONS

Morphology

The medium-size densely spiny neuron, so called because of its appearance in Golgi preparation (i.e. medium-size perikaryon, spine free primary dendrites and densely spiny secondary and higher order dendrites) is the most frequently impregnated neuron-type in Golgi preparations of the striatum (17, 22) and probably does in fact represent the majority of striatal neurons. Not only are they the most common type of striatal neuron but they are also the major type of striatal projection neuron sending their axons to the pallidal complex and/or the substantia nigra. (10, 34) The axons of these neurons, before leaving the striatum, give rise to extensive local collaterals that form bouton-like swellings, which, on examination in the electron microscope of Golgi-impregnated or horseradish peroxidase-filled examples, have been shown to form typical symmetrical synaptic specialization. The postsynaptic target of these terminals, that can be identified with most certainty, are other neurons that possess spines and are therefore probably also medium-size densely spiny neurons.(32,38)

Putative Transmitters

Putative transmitters that have been ascribed to medium-size densely spiny neurons include GABA, substance P, and enkephalin or a related peptide. By combining Golgi-impregnation with immunocytochemistry for the putative transmitters, populations of medium-size densely spiny neurons have been identified that contain substance P or met. enkephalin (4). These observations are consistent with results of several experimental approaches that suggest these peptides are present in striatal output pathways.(See 18, 20) Neurochemical analysis combined with pathway lesions are also consistent with the presence of GABA in the striatonigral pathway and therefore presumably medium-size densely spiny neurons. Direct morphological evidence of this is not yet available although populations of striatal neurons immunoreactive for GAD (glutamate decarboxylase), the synthetic enzyme for GABA, are similar in light microscopic morphology to medium-size densely spiny neurons. (9, 28). It is of interest that at least in a subpopulation of medium-sized striatal neurons GAD and enkephalin coexist (1). The possibility also exists that medium-size densely spiny neurons contain taurine or a related substance since neurons characterized by Golgi-impregnation or by the retrograde transport of horseradish peroxidase from the substantia nigra accumulate exogenous radiolabelled taurine (13 and Clarke unpublished).

Synaptic Input

In order to understand how the release of transmitters from these neurons is affected by other neurotransmitters we need to know the origin and chemical characteristics of their afferent synaptic input and, just as importantly, the spatial relationships upon the neurons of afferent synapses of different origin or chemistry. Electron microscopic analysis of Golgi-impregnated neurons, HRP-injected neurons or neurons that were both Golgi-impregnated and retrogradely labelled with HRP from the substantia nigra, reveals that the synaptic input can be divided into two broad morphological categories, those forming asymmetrical synaptic specializations and those forming symmetrical specializations (19, 34). These two types have distinct distributions; asymmetrical specializations only occur on dendritic spines while symmetrical specializations occur on all parts of the neuron but mainly on the perikarya, proximal dendritic shafts and dendritic spines. Relatively few synapses occur on the shafts of dendrites in their more distal regions i.e. the spiny region. The chemistry and origin of many of these synapses has been characterized by combining Golgi-impregnation (with or without the retrograde transport of HRP from the substantia nigra) with anterograde synaptic degeneration or immunocytochemistry for transmitters or transmitter markers.

Asymmetrical Input (Cortical)
At least some of the terminals that form asymmetrical specializations with the spines of medium-size densely spiny neurons are derived from the cortex. Examination in the electron microscope of Golgi-impregnated medium-size densely spiny neurons that were also retrogradely labelled with HRP from the SN from rats that had also received multiple electrolytic lesions of the cortex revealed the presence of degenerating synaptic input to these neurons (32). All the degenerating terminals found in contact with the neurons made asymmetrical synaptic specializations with dendritic spines and therefore in the more distal regions of the neurons. Thus one of the targets of corticostriatal fibres are the spines of striatonigral neurons. A large body of evidence supports the hypothesis that the

transmitter of these terminals is an excitatory amino acid , probably glutamate (See 20). One could predict therefore that glutamate will affect the release of the transmitter(s) present in the spiny neurons. However, these terminals contact relatively distal parts of the neuron; the effect of cortical stimulation on the output of the cell will be dependent, among other factors, on the activity of synapses located more proximally.

Symmetrical Input

Three catergories of terminals that form symmetrical synaptic specializations in contact with medium-size densely spiny neurons, have so far been identified. These are 1) tyrosine hydroxylase-immunoreactive terminals i.e. dopaminergic terminals from the SN, 2) GAD-immunoreactive terminals i.e. GABAergic terminals and 3) substance P-immunoreactive terminals.

Tyrosine hydroxylase-immunoreactive terminals. The studies of Freund, Powell and Smith (19) have demonstrated that Golgi-impregnated medium-size densely spiny neurons, identified as striatonigral by the retrograde transport of HRP, receive symmetrical synaptic input from terminals immunoreactive for tyrosine hydroxylase (TH). One of the most interesting points about their observations was the pattern of the dopaminergic input to the neurons. A high proportion of the immunoreactive terminals (approx. 60%) made synaptic contact with necks of dendritic spines and each postsynaptic spine was always associated with another, non-immunoreactive, input at the head of the spine which formed asymmetrical synaptic specializations. Most of the other immunoreative terminals made contact with dendritic shafts but most of these were close to the point of origin of spines. At least some of the TH-positive boutons occur on the necks of spines that also receive input (asymmetrical) from the cortex, as shown by the anterograde degeneration study of Bouyer et al. (8). Thus one site of interaction between the dopaminergic input and the cortical input to the striatum is on the postsynaptic structure i.e. dendritic spines of striatonigral neurons. Freund et al (19) have speculated that dopamine will have a very selective effect on the cortical input to the spiny neurons, perhaps blocking in some way, the cortical input to the neurons. Interpretations of some pharmacological data and electrophysiological data are consistent with these suggestions (See Arbuthnott, this volume)

GAD-immunoreactive terminals. By combining Golgi-impregnation with GAD immunocytochemistry, terminals that possess the capability to synthesize GABA have been shown to make direct synaptic contact with medium-size densely spiny neurons. The terminals made symmetrical synaptic contact with the perikarya, proximal dendritic shafts (Figure 1) and to a lesser extent the distal dendritic shafts of Golgi-impregnated medium-size densely spiny neurons. Only one terminal was found in contact with a dendritic spine. (5) The distribution of the immunoreactive terminals was consistent with the overall distribution of the post synaptic targets of 'randomly identified' GAD-containing terminals; most were in contact with perikarya and dendritic shafts and only about 6% were in contact with spines.

Substance P-immunoreactive terminals. The combination of substance P immunocytochemistry and Golgi impregnation or the retrograde transport of horseradish peroxidase from the substantia nigra, has shown that Golgi-impregnated medium-size densely spiny neurons as well as identified striatonigral neurons (Figure 2) receive direct synaptic input from substance P-containing boutons. The distribution of the boutons was very similar to that of the GAD-containing terminals; most were in contact with perikarya and proximal dendritic shafts while only few were in contact with distal shafts and only rarely were contacts made with spines.

The origin of the GABAergic and the substance P boutons are unclear; they may be derived from extrinsic sources and/or local neurons. The GABA terminals may be derived from the non-dopaminergic part of the striatonigral pathway or from the pallidostriatal pathway (for references see 5), similarily substance P boutons may be derived from the thalamus (35). However there are at least two types of GABAergic neurons in the striatum (for references see 2 and 5) and at least two types of substance P-containing neurons (6), that give rise to local terminals. The morphology of both types of immunoreactive terminals are similar to those of identified medium-size densely spiny neurons, it is therefore likely that a significant proportion are derived from local neurons.

These results suggest firstly, that the two known extrinsic inputs to medium-size densely spiny neurons occur on the more distal parts of the neuron which represents a site of transmitter interaction on the postsynaptic neuron and may represent a site of 'self integration', in a very selective manner, of extrinsic inputs without much influence of local neurons. This may also be the case for some of the other extrinsic inputs to the striatum, if indeed they make contact with spiny neurons, since ultrastructural analysis has shown that thalamostriatal terminals and 5HT-immunoreactive terminals make asymmetrical synaptic specializations, i.e. the type that only occurs on the spines. (23, 24, 30) Second, local input to spiny neurons (probably from other spiny neurons) occurs predominantly in the more proximal regions of the neurons. Integrated extrinsic information coming from the distal regions of the neurons will therefore be influenced in a much more non-selective manner by local inputs in the more proximal regions of the neuron. The effect of glutamate, for instance, on the output of a spiny neuron will depend not only on the activity of the glutamate-containing terminals but also the activity of the other, more proximally located, afferent synapses to the neuron, including dopaminergic terminals and terminals containing GAD or substance P. Thus in order to have a complete understanding of the possible interactions of

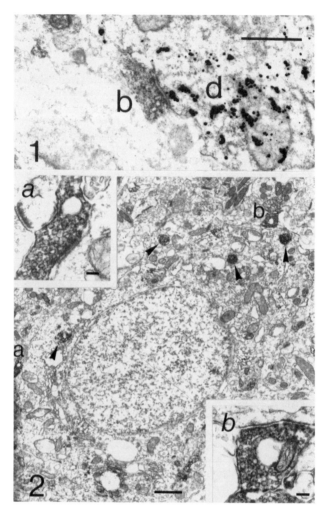

Figure 1. An electron micrograph of a GAD-immunoreactive bouton (b) in symmetrical contact with the dendritic shaft (d) of a Golgi-impregnated medium-size densely spiny neuron, that was first identified in the light microscope and then examined in the electron microscope. The neuron was identified in the electron microscope by the electron dense secondary Golgi deposit. Scale: 0.5µm

Figure 2. Low power electron micrograph of a striatonigral neuron identified by the reaction product (arrow heads) formed by horseradish peroxidase retrogradely transported from the substantia nigra. The neuron is postsynaptic to two substance P-immunoreactive terminals (symmetrical specializations) (a & b) shown at higher power in the insets (a & b). Scale: 1µm; a and b, 0.1µm

transmitters at the single cell level it is important to know not only the characteristics of individual afferent synapses but also the spatial relationships or the pattern of the terminals on the target neuron.

In addition to the possibility that other striatal afferents make contact with spiny neurons indirect evidence suggests that other types of local neuron also make synaptic contact with them; terminals immunoreactive for enkephalin, somatostatin and choline acetyltransferase have all been shown to make synaptic contact with neurons that possess the ultrastructural characteristics of medium-size densely spiny neurons. (14, 15, 16, 33, 36, 37) Further work is required to confirm these observations and to establish their exact location on the neurons.

CHOLINERGIC INTERNEURONS

With the advent of specific antibodies against choline acetyltransferase (ChAT) (26) it has become possible to morphologically characterise cholinergic neurons and their synaptic input. The combination of ChAT immunocytochemistry with Golgi-impregnation has demonstrated that cholinergic neurons are a type of large aspiny neuron that have long dendrites extending up to one millimetre from the cell body and have often been referred to as the giant neuron of the striatum. (7) They are of the same class of large neuron that stains intensely for acetylcholinesterase (3). Neurochemical evidence, as well as the fact that the axons of Golgi-impregnated neurons of the same type as stain for ChAT are typical of interneurons, suggests that, at least in the rat, they are intrinsic to the striatum. The synaptic input to cholinergic neurons is of at least four types; two types that form symmetrical synaptic specializations which account for most of the contacts on proximal dendrites and perikarya and two types of asymmetrical specializations, one of which possesses dense sub-junctional bodies and has been found in proximal regions of the neuron. The other type of asymmetrical synapse occurs more frequently in the more distal parts of the dendrites, where both symmetrical and asymmetrical synaptic specializations are observed.

Since the cholinergic neurons are, in all probablity, interneurons and there is no known cholinergic input to the striatum, then any pharmacological or behavioural data relating to cholinergic parameters is most likely a consequence of the activity of these neurons. As stated above cholinergic neurons are anatomically distinct and can be recognised, with a fair degree of certainty, even without histochemical stains. Anatomical study of these neurons therefore offers a unique opportunity to test pharmacological data and to provide information as to which transmitter substances may affect the activity of cholinergic neurons and the output of acetylcholine.

Many striatal transmitters have been shown to affect the turnover or the release of acetylcholine: dopamine, GABA and 5HT inhibit the turnover or release of acetylcholine, while glutamate (derived from the cortex) stimulates them. (For references see 12, 25). It is unclear where these substances are acting upon the neurons; pharmacological data would suggest that dopamine acts on cholinergic terminals while the effect of GABA may at least in part be an indirect action on cortical terminals since the inhibitory effect of GABA is attenuated by destruction of the corticostriatal pathway (31). We have begun a series of experiments in an attempt to characterize, morphologically, the types of boutons afferent to the cholinergic neuron.

GAD- and substance P-positive input to large neurons.   In material incubated to reveal GAD or substance P immunoreactivity and post-fixed with osmium for electron microscopy, large or giant neurons are often clearly visible. In the light microscope, the perikarya and proximal dendrites of these large cells are invariably associated with immunoreactive punctate structures. Electron microscopic analysis of these neurons reveals that the ultrastructure and types and pattern of afferent synaptic boutons are similar to those of identified cholinergic neurons. The immunoreactive punctate structures are found to be axonal boutons that form symmetrical synaptic specializations with the cholinergic-like neurons. These observations suggest that cholinergic neurons receive direct synaptic input from terminals containing substance P and from terminals that can synthesize GABA. At least part of the inhibitory effect of GABA on cholinergic neurons is therefore probably a direct effect on the cell body and proximal dendrites. One explanation for the attenuation of the effect of GABA by cortical lesions may be that the effect of GABA is greatest when the neuron is under cortical drive that originates in more distal regions of the neuron. Since substance P-containing terminals also make contact with large cholinergic-like neurons one can predict that substance P will affect the activity of cholinergic neurons or the turnover or output of ACh and that any effect will be dependent on the state of the corticostriatal pathway. However, one report describes no effect of substance P on the turnover of ACh in the striatum despite the fact that turnover was affected in other brain regions. (27)

As with the medium-size densely spiny neurons, the origin of these two inputs is uncertain, however one can speculate that they are both derived from local GABAergic and substance P-containing neurons.

The criteria for identification of cholinergic neurons in these experiments were indirect; direct evidence of the chemical characteristics of afferents to cholinergic neurons can only be obtained by the application of double immunocytochemical techniques.

Substance P-positive input to identified cholinergic neurons. The suggestion that substance P-containing terminals make direct synaptic contact with cholinergic neurons has been confirmed by using a double immunocytochemical procedure to identify the chemical nature of both the pre and post synaptic structures. (21). Sections of rat striatum were incubated first to reveal substance P immunoreactivity by the peroxidase anti-peroxidase

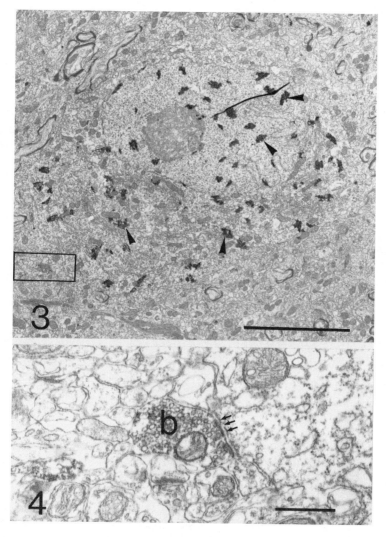

Figure 3. Electron micrograph of a choline acetyltransferase-immunoreactive neuron. The immunoreactivity was localized using benzidine dihydrochloride as the substrate for the peroxidase reaction, some of the granules of which are indicated by arrows. The section was also incubated for substance P-immunoreactivity but using diaminobenzidine as the substrate, a substance P-containing bouton (boxed area) is shown at higher power in figure 4. Scale: 5μm.

Figure 4. High power electron micrograph of the substance P-immunoreactive bouton (b) shown in figure 3. The bouton is in symmetrical synaptic contact (arrow) with the choline acetyltransferase-immunoreactive neuron. Scale: 0.5μm.

procedure and using diaminobenzidine as the substrate and then for ChAT immunoreactivity but this time using benzidine dihyrochloride as the substrate. The two substrates produce reaction products that are distinct in both the light and electron microscopes. Electron microscopic analysis revealed that the perikarya and proximal dendrites of cholinergic neurons received direct synaptic input from terminals immunoreactive for substance P. (Figures 3 and 4)

Experiments are in progress to confirm the GABAergic input to identified cholinergic neurons and to determine whether dopamine-containing, 5HT-containing and cortical terminals make direct synaptic contact with cholinergic neurons, and if so, to determine the spatial relationships of the afferents on their target neuron.

Summary. The studies we have described on two types of striatal neuron have shown that the interactions between transmitters are spatially organised at the level of an individual neuron type. In order to draw functionally meaningful conclusions, it is now clearly necessary to take into account the location of transmitter-specific boutons on different parts of a neuron. These morphological studies therefore lay the basis of biophysical, physiological and pharmacological studies that will give further insights into the complexity of information flow through the striatum.

REFERENCES

1. Aronin, N., DiFiglia, M., Graveland, G.A., Scharwtz, W.J. and Wu, J.-Y. (1984): Brain Res., 300:376-380.
2. Bolam, J.P., Clarke, D.J., Smith, A.D. and Somogyi, P. (1983): J. Comp.Neurol., 213:121-134.
3. Bolam, J.P., Ingham, C.A. and Smith, A.D. (1984): Neuroscience, 12:687-709.
4. Bolam, J.P., Izzo, P.N. and Graybiel, A.M. (1985): Neurosci. Letts. Suppl. 22:S281.
5. Bolam, J.P., Powell, J.F., Wu, J.-Y. and Smith, A.D. (1985): J. Comp. Neurol., 237:1-20.
6. Bolam, J.P., Somogyi, P., Takagi, H., Fodor, I. and Smith A.D. (1983): J. Neurocytol., 12:325-344.
7. Bolam, J.P., Wainer, B.H. and Smith, A.D. (1984): Neuroscience, 12:711-718.
8. Bouyer, J.J., Park, D.H., Joh, T.H. and Pickel, V.M. (1984): Brain Res., 302:267-275.
9. Bradley, R.H., Kitai, S.T. and Wu, J.-Y. (1983): Soc. Neurosci. Abstr., 9:658.
10. Chang, H.T., Wilson, C.J. and Kitai, S.T. (1981): Science, 213:915-918.

11. Chang, H.T., Wilson, C.J. and Kitai, S.T. (1982): J. Comp. Neurol., 208:107-126.
12. Chesselet, M.-F. (1984): Neuroscience, 12:347-375.
13. Clarke, D.J., Smith, A.D. and Bolam, J.P. (1983): Brain Res., 289:342-348.
14. DiFiglia, M. and Aronin, N. (1982). J. Neurosci., 2:1267-1274.
15. DiFiglia, M. and Aronin, N. (1984). Neurosci. Letts., 50:325-331.
16. DiFiglia, M., Aronin, N. and Martin, J.B. (1982): J. Neurosci., 2:303-320.
17. DiFiglia, M., Pasik, P. and Pasik, T. (1976): Brain Res., 114:245-256.
18. Dray, A. (1979): Neuroscience, 4:1407-1439.
19. Freund, T.F., Powell, J.F. and Smith, A.D. (1984): Neuroscience, 13:1189-1215.
20. Graybiel, A.M. and Ragsdale, C.W. (1983): In: Chemical Neuroanatomy, edited by P.C. Emson, pp.427-504. Raven Press, New York.
21. Izzo, P.N., Wainer, B.H., Rye, D.B., Levey, A.I. and Bolam, J.P. (1985): Neurosci. Letts. Suppl., 22:S410 .
22. Kemp, J.M. and Powell, T.P.S. (1971): Philos. Trans. R. Soc. B., 262:383-401.
23. Kemp, J.M. and Powell, T.P.S. (1971): Philos. Trans. R. Soc. B., 262:413-427.
24. Kemp, J.M. and Powell, T.P.S. (1971): Philos. Trans. R. Soc. B., 262:429-439.
25. Lehman, J. and Langer, S.Z. (1983): Neuroscience, 10:1105-1120.
26. Levey, A.I., Armstrong, D.M., Atweh, S.F., Terry, R.D. and Wainer, B.H. (1983): J. Neurosci., 3:1-9.
27. Malthe-Sorensen, D. and Wood, P. (1979): In: The Cholinergic Synapse. Progress in Brain Res. vol.49, edited by S. Tucek, pp.486-487. Elsevier.
28. Oertel, W.H. and Mugnaini, E. (1983): Soc. Neurosci. Abstr., 9:14.
29. Palkovits, M. (1984): Prog. Neurobiol., 23:151-189.
30. Pasik, P., Pasik, T., Holstein, G.R. and Pecci Saavedra, J. (1984): In: The Basal Ganglia structure and Function, edited by J.S. McKenzie, R.E. Kemm and L.N. Wilcock, pp.115-129. Plenum Press, New York and London.
31. Scatton, B. and Bartholini, G. (1980): Brain Res., 200:174-178.
32. Somogyi, P., Bolam, J.P. and Smith, A.D. (1981): J. Comp. Neurol., 195:567-584.
33. Somogyi, P., Priestly, J.V., Cuello, A.C., Smith, A.D. and Takagi, H. (1982): J. Neurocytol., 11:779-807.
34. Somogyi, P. and Smith, A.D. (1979): Brain Res., 178:3-15.
35. Sugimoto, T., Takada, M., Kaneko, T. and Mizuno, N. (1984): Brain Res., 323:181-184.

36. Takagi, H., Somogyi, P., Somogyi, J. and Smith, A.D. (1983):
    J. Comp. Neurol., 214:1-16.
37. Wainer, B.H., Bolam, J.P., Freund, T.F., Henderson, Z.F.,
    Totterdell, S. and Smith, A.D. (1984): Brain Res.,
    308:69-76.
38. Wilson, C.J. and Groves, P.M. (1980): J. Comp. Neurol.,
    194:599-615.

Neurotransmitter Interactions in the Basal Ganglia, edited by M. Sandler et al.
Raven Press, New York © 1987.

ULTRASTRUCTURAL DISTRIBUTION OF MU OPIOID RECEPTORS
IN RAT NEOSTRIATUM

Edith Hamel and Alain Beaudet

Laboratory of Neuroanatomy, Montreal Neurological
Institute, 3801 University Street, Montréal, Québec,
Canada H3A 2B4

When opioid receptors were first demonstrated in mammalian brain, the neostriatum was identified as the cerebral region containing the highest levels of these binding sites (40). Shortly thereafter, the striatum and various other brain structures were shown to contain Met- and Leu-enkephalin (60) the first endogenous opioid substances to be characterized. The fact that the enkephalins could be released from striatal slices by depolarization (25) and could influence motor activity and striatal dopamine metabolism (5,33,39) strongly suggested a role for opioid peptides in the control of striatal neuronal activity.

Since these early reports, several observations have emphasized the importance of opioid substances in striatal function. Three of the opioid receptor subtypes so far identified, namely μ, δ and k sites, are represented in the striatum where they exhibit specific and characteristic distributional patterns (19,27,34,43). Enkephalins and dynorphins, two of the three families of opioid peptides present in mammalian CNS (30), are widely distributed in neurones and fibres located within the neostriatum (41,50-52,55-57). In addition, the enzyme which appears to be involved in terminating the action of opioid enkephalin peptides, the neutral endopeptidase designated as "enkephalinase", has been localized in rat brain and is particularly concentrated in the neostriatum(53-54).

Despite numerous attempts to identify the cellular localization of opioid receptors in the neostriatum, little is still known concerning the precise site(s) of action of striatal opioid peptides. Biochemical investigations have shown that nuclear, microsomal and synaptosomal subcellular fractions all contain substantial amounts of opioid binding sites (18,40,47).

In addition, selective lesion experiments have suggested that opioid receptors might be present on intrinsic neostriatal neurones, as well as on meso-striatal dopaminergic and corticostriate axon terminals (12,36,42,45). However, lesion studies provide only indirect information on the cellular localization of the receptors; in addition, the interpretation of the results is complicated by the occurrence of trans-synaptic degeneration of post-synaptic dendrites, documented after decortication or lesion of nigrostriatal afferents (24).

In an attempt to reach a better understanding of the mode of action of opioid peptides in neostriatum, the distribution of selectively labeled μ-opioid binding sites was examined by light and electron microscopic radioautography in sections of rat caudate-putamen. Our results indicate that the majority of labeled opioid binding sites is associated with axodendritic, axoaxonic and axosomatic neuronal membrane interfaces, an observation compatible with both a post- and a pre- synaptic localization of μ-opioid receptors in neostriatum. The present data further suggest that striatal opioid peptides act chiefly on receptors located on non-junctional neuronal membranes.

METHODOLOGY

Mu opioid receptors were selectively labeled in vitro, using ^{125}I-FK 33-824 (Tyr-D-Ala-Gly-MePhe-Met(o)ol; ^{125}I-FK), a non-degradable met-enkephalin analog (9,10,46). The radioautographic detection of labeled binding sites was achieved after chemical cross-link of the bound ^{125}I-FK to tissue proteins through its free primary amino group. For this purpose, glutaraldehyde (4%) was used as bifunctional cross-linking agent. All binding experiments (1nM ^{125}I-FK in 0.05 M Tris-HCl containing 0.25 M sucrose, pH 7.4) were performed on vibratome-cut sections prefixed with a solution that contained low concentrations of aldehydes in order to preserve the fine structure of the tissue. The proportion and repartition of non-specific binding sites were determined in sections incubated in the presence of 1 μM naloxone or 1 μM non-radioactive FK. The details of the method have been extensively described in previous reports (22,23). At the light microscopic level, the distribution and number of the total and non-specific binding sites were evaluated by grain scoring in bright field photomicrographs from both patches and matrix areas. At the electron microscopic level, the distribution of ^{125}I-FK labeled opioid binding sites was analyzed within patches of high labeling densities using 50% probability circles (diameter = 3.4 x half-distance (HD); HD = 90 nm (48,59)) in sections incubated with ^{125}I-FK alone (total binding) as well as in sections incubated in the presence of 1 μM naloxone (non-specific binding). The distribution of specific binding sites was derived from grain counts performed in sections incubated with ^{125}I-FK alone and corrected for non-specific binding according to the distribution of silver grains in sections incubated in the presence of naloxone.

RESULTS

Localization of opioid receptors at the light microscopic level.

Light microscopic examination of radioautographs from sections (1 µm-thick) incubated with ^{125}I-FK alone revealed a heterogeneous distribution of the silver grains characterized by the presence of "patches" of high labeling densities superimposed over a moderately labeled matrix, as expected from the selective labeling of µ-opioid binding sites (19,27). Both within and outside patches, the majority of silver grains was detected over the neuropil (70.9% vs 68.3% ; see Figs. 1a and 1b, respectively). In some cases, the grains appeared associated with the cytoplasmic membrane of large proximal dendrites and neuronal cell bodies (Figs. 1a,b). A smaller proportion of silver grains overlaid myelinated fibre bundles (15.3% in patches vs 20.3% in matrix) and nerve cell bodies (13.1% vs 9.3%). In sections incubated in the presence of 1 µM naloxone (non-specific

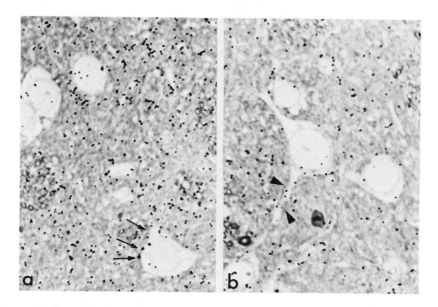

Figure 1. Light microscopic radioautographs from 1 µm-thick sections of rat neostriatum after incubation with ^{125}I-FK. Localization of opioid binding sites within a patch (a) and in the matrix area (b). Note the presence of numerous silver grains over the neuropil and the relative sparing of nerve cell bodies and myelinated fibre bundles. Some silver grains directly overlay the cytoplasmic membrane of large proximal dendrites (arrowheads) and neuronal cell bodies (arrows). X 1650.

binding), the labeling was more sparse, but similarly predominated over the neuropil (68.3% of the grains). Both radioactivity measurements and grain counts indicated that these sections contained 80% less radioactivity than those incubated with ^{125}I-FK alone (total binding).

Both neuropil and nerve cell bodies were significantly more densely labeled within patches (31.0 $\pm$ 2.6 and 19.3 $\pm$ 2.9 grains/1000μm^2, respectively) than in the intervening matrix (9.3 $\pm$ 0.7 and 3.0 $\pm$ 0.6 grains/1000μm^2, respectively). This difference was particularly striking in the case of nerve cell bodies (see above).

Localization of opioid receptors at the ultrastructural level.

Specifically labeled ^{125}I-FK binding sites were mainly associated with apposed neuronal structures (>75%, shared grains; Table I). The same proportion as in light microscopic preparations overlaid nerve cell bodies (20.5%, exclusive grains; Table I). Finally, an even smaller fraction was ascribed to non-neuronal or unidentified neuronal structures (3.9%, "others", Table I). A line source analysis carried out on 100 silver grains overlying two adjacent neuronal structures indicated that 70% of shared grains were within one half distance of either one of the apposed membranes, suggesting that radioactive sources were associated with the plasma membranes themselves. However, because of limitations inherent to the radioautographic technique, it was not possible to determine to which of the apposed membranes the radioactive sources were actually linked. Shared grains were mainly distributed over axodendritic, axoaxonic and axosomatic neuronal interfaces.

More than half of striatal opioid binding sites were associated with axodendritic appositions (Table I). These appositions mainly involved small axon terminals (0.75 μm in diameter) containing numerous small, round, electrolucent vesicles and rare large agranular vesicles. Their dendritic counterparts were mainly dendritic branches (Fig. 2a) but also included dendritic shafts as well as dendritic spines. A large proportion of labeled dendritic profiles exhibited slender spinous projections; others showed none and thus presumably corresponded to the smooth dendrites of striatal aspiny neurones (6,16). In most cases (45.8%), no membrane specialization was present at the site of apposition, though occasionally (7.1%), a well-defined synaptic complex was included within the resolution circle. When present, synaptic specializations were mostly asymmetric (5.8%) and established on dendritic spines (4.0%, Fig. 2b). The rare labeled symmetric synapses (1.4%) were exclusively observed on dendritic branches. A few dendrites exhibited multiple sites of labeling (junctional and/or non-junctional) along their plasma membrane, a pattern highly suggestive of a dendritic localization of the labeled receptors.

TABLE 1 – DISTRIBUTION OF HYPOTHETICAL AND REAL GRAINS IN 125I–FK
LABELLED STRIATAL SECTIONS

Included within 50 % probability circle	Hypothetical	Real (non-specific)	Real (specific)
Single structures (exclusive grains)			
Nerve cell bodies	23.3	12.5	13.1
Axon terminals	12.1	10.7	1.5
Dendrites	18.7	19.3	5.9
Apposed structures (shared grains)			
Axon/Dendrite			
Synaptic complex not included	12.7	10.3	45.8
Synaptic complex included	3.1	1.2	7.1
Axon/Axon	9.5	13.4	17.6
Axon/Soma	1.0	1.4	3.2
Dendrite/Dendrite	6.1	7.0	1.9
Others	13.5	24.2	3.9
Number of grains counted	10,039	499	1,961

Distribution of specific and non-specific ^{125}I–FK labeled opioid binding sites (real grains) in sections from rat striatum. The data are expressed as percentages and correspond to the mean of five different experiments. Silver grains were ascribed to underlying cellular structures using a 50% probability circle (see text). The hypothetical distribution was generated by means of a transparent overlay displaying a regular array of resolution circles. X^2 analyses showed that the three distributions were significantly different ($p < 0.005$).

Axoaxonic appositions accounted for the second largest source of striatal μ-opioid binding sites (17.6%, Table I). Such appositions involved either two axon terminals or one axon terminal and one or more unmyelinated axonal processes (Fig. 2). The axon terminals were similar to those involved in labeled axodendritic appositions. Synaptic specializations were never visible at the site of contact. In many instances, however, one of the terminals was seen in synaptic contact with a dendritic profile, usually a dendritic spine (Fig. 2c).

A small proportion of striatal opioid binding sites was associated with axosomatic appositions (3.2%, Table I). Recipient neurones were generally of medium size (12-22 μm in diameter) and possessed a large round or ovoid nucleus with no or very little indentation, and a cytoplasm rather poor in organelles. These were identified as spiny type I neurones according to previous cytoarchitectonic descriptions of rat neostriatum (6,16). In most cases, no synaptic density was observed at the interface between the axon terminal and the neuronal perikarya.

Exclusive grains were mainly found over neuronal perikarya (13%) and dendrites (5.9%, Table I). The labeling was found over the cytoplasm, nucleus, nuclear membrane as well as over a number of intra-cytoplasmic organelles.

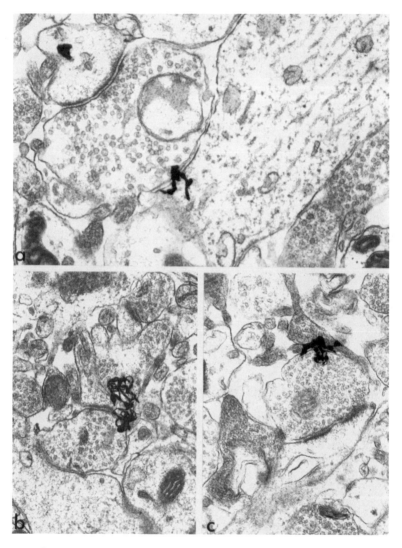

Figure 2. Electron microscopic radioautographs of μ-opioid binding sites labeled in rat neostriatum. The labeling is detected as stray silver grains overlying the plasma membranes of two apposed neuronal structures. a, Silver grain associated with a non-junctional axodendric apposition. X 36,400. b, Labeled junctional axodendritic contact; one of the silver grains overlies an asymmetric synaptic complex between an axon terminal and a dendritic spine. X 26,000. c, Axoaxonic binding site; the silver grain overlies the apposition between at least two axonal processes. Note that one of the axon terminals is in synaptic contact with a dendritic spine. X 26,000.

DISCUSSION

The present radioautographic study demonstrates that the vast majority of μ-opioid binding sites labeled with ^{125}I-FK in rat neostriatum are associated with neuronal membrane interfaces. Close to 60% of the labeled binding sites are associated with axodendritic and axosomatic contacts established predominantly on medium spiny neurones. Due to limitations in the resolution of the radioautographic technique, it is not possible to determine on which of the apposed membranes the receptors are actually localized. Nevertheless, the presence of several binding sites along the plasma membrane of certain dendrites and perikarya strongly argue for a dendritic or "post-synaptic" localization of at least some of the labeled receptors. A localization on the dendrites and perikarya of neostriatal neurones (but also on local circuit axons) would be compatible with the decrease in striatal opioid receptors reported after destruction of intrastriatal neurones by kainic acid (8,12,36,49). It is interesting to recall, in this context, that intrastriatal kainic acid also induces a drop of opioid binding sites in the globus pallidus and substantia nigra (1), presumably through lesion of striatofugal medium spiny neurones.

The high proportion (17.6%) of specific binding sites labeled at the level of axoaxonic appositions is consistent, on the other hand, with the presence of opioid receptors on the plasma membranes of axonal processes. In view of a recent report (17) showing that the terminal fields of pre-limbic cortical projections fill in the striatal patches of opioid receptors, and that enkephalin-immunoreactive terminals are directly apposed to cortico-striate axons (7), it is tempting to speculate that some of the receptors labeled in the present study are located on corticostriate projections. The substantial decrease in opioid receptors observed after cerebral decortication (12) supports this hypothesis. A significant proportion of ^{125}I-FK axoaxonic binding sites could also be associated with nigrostriate dopaminergic axon terminals, whose selective cytotoxic destruction has been shown to result in a significant loss of opioid receptors in rat neostriatum (36,42,45,49). Such pre-synaptic receptors could account for some of the effects of opioid peptides on the metabolism and release of dopamine in the neostriatum (11). Finally, a pre-synaptic localization of opioid receptors on serotonergic axon terminals has been invoked to explain the decrease in opioid receptors observed after destruction of mesencephalic raphé nuclei (37).

A major finding from the present work is that the majority of labeled opioid binding sites are located on membrane appositions lacking the morphological specializations that normally characterize synaptic junctions. Such lack of correlation between labeled binding sites and synapses was much less apparent in the case of other neurotransmitter receptors so far localized at the ultrastructural level in rat CNS (2,3,28,31,32,35).

Nevertheless, the vast majority of ^{125}I-FK-labeled binding sites was associated with neuronal interfaces involving one or several axonal processes (more than 90% of the labeled appositions included an axonal process) suggesting that the labeled sites correspond to a functional form of the receptors. Whether the labeled axons are themselves the site of storage and release of the endogenous ligand or whether they contain another neurotransmitter whose release – or effects – are modulated by opiates remains to be determined. Several lines of evidence suggest that the enkephalins or other opioid peptides derived from pro-enkephalin may normally interact with the labeled binding sites (58). Indeed, most of these peptides show moderate to high affinity for the μ-opioid receptors (44) and are contained within axon terminals that appear to be concentrated, in both rat and cat neostriatum, within patches of high μ-opioid receptor densities (17,20,38). Interestingly, in rat neostriatum, enkephalin immunoreactive terminals exhibit ultrastructural characteristics that compare reasonably well with those of axon terminals labeled in the present study, suggesting that enkephalins might be released by terminals that either possess or are immediately adjacent to ^{125}I-FK labeled opioid binding sites. Enkephalin terminals were shown, in particular, to establish asymmetric contacts with dendritic spines and both asymmetric and symmetric contacts with dendritic branches and never to engage in axoaxonic synapses (41,51). Moreover, a large number reportedly failed to exhibit synaptic differentiations in single thin sections (41). Enkephalins could obviously also be released from axon terminals distinct from the labeled ones and diffuse in tissue over a relatively large distance to act on a widespread population of receptors. Such a mechanism has already been postulated, on the basis of radioautographic, immunocytochemical and/or electrophysiological evidence for opioids as well as for other neuropeptides and the monoamines in both central and peripheral nervous systems (4,13-15,21,26,29). In any event, the present data strongly suggest that opioid peptides in neostriatum may exert their effects in the absence of membrane specialization, via non-junctional receptors.

ACKNOWLEDGEMENTS

We thank K. Leonard and C. Hodge for technical assistance, Dr. M. Dennis for his help with the iodination of the peptide and M.-L. Pernelet for typing the manuscript. FK 33-824 was kindly provided by Dr. D. Roemer (Sandoz, Basel). This work was supported by a fellowship (E.H.), a scholarship (A.B.) and grant MA-7366 from the MRC of Canada. E.H. is now with the Cerebral Circulation and Metabolism Group, Laboratoires d'Etudes et de Recherches Synthélabo (L.E.R.S.), 31, ave P.V. Couturier, Bagneux, 92220 – France.

REFERENCES

1. Abou-Khalil, B., Young, A.B. and Penney, J.B. (1984): Brain Res. 323: 21-29.
2. Arimatsu, Y., Seto, A. and Amano, T. (1978): Brain Res. 231: 1-17.
3. Arluison, M., Martres, M.-P. and Sokoloff, P. (1983): J. Neural. Transm. Suppl. 18: 9-24.
4. Barker, J.L. (1978): Neurosci. Res. Prog. Bull. 16: 535-553.
5. Biggio, G., Casa, M., Corda, M., DiBello, C. and Gessa, G.L. (1978): Science 200: 552-554.
6. Bishop, G.A., Chang, H.T. and Kitai, S.T. (1982) Neuroscience 7: 179-191.
7. Bouyer, J.J., Miller, R.J. and Pickel, V.M. (1984): Regulatory Peptides 8: 105-115.
8. Bowen, W.D., Pert, C.B. and Pert, A. (1982): Life Sci. 31: 1679-1682.
9. Chang, K.-J., Cooper, B.R., Hazum, E. and Cuatrecasas, P. (1979): Mol. Pharmacol. 16: 91-104.
10. Chang, K.-J. and Cuatrecasas, P. (1979): J. Biol. Chem. 54: 2610-2618.
11. Chesselet, M.-F., Chéramy, A., Reisine, T.D., Lubetzki, C., Desban, M. and Glowinski, J. (1983): Brain Res. 258: 229-242.
12. Childers, S.R., Schwarcz, R., Coyle, J.T. and Snyder, S.H. (1978): In: Adv. Biochem. Pharmacol. 18: 161-173.
13. Cuello, A.C. (1983): Brit. Med. Bull. 39: 11-16.
14. Cuello, A.C. (1983): Fedn. Proc. 42: 2912-2922.
15. Descarries, L., Beaudet, A. and Watkins, K.C. (1975): Brain Res. 100: 563-588.
16. Dimova, R., Vuillet. J. and Seite, R. (1980): Neuroscience 5: 1581-1596.
17. Gerfen, C.R. (1984): Nature 311: 461-464.
18. Glasel, J.A., Venn, R.F. and Barnard, E.A. (1980): Biochem. Biophys. Res. Commun. 95: 263-268.
19. Goodman, R.R., Snyder, S.H., Kuhar, M.J. and Young, W.S. (1980): Proc. Natl. Acad. Sci. USA 77: 6239-6243.
20. Graybiel, A.M. and Chesselet, M.-F. (1984): Proc. Natl. Acad. Sci. USA 81: 7980-7984.
21. Guy, J., Vaudry, H. and Pelletier, G. (1982): Brain Res. 239: 265-270.
22. Hamel, E. and Beaudet, A. (1984): J. Electron Microsc. Tech. 1: 317-329.
23. Hamel, E. and Beaudet, A. (1984): Nature 312: 155-157.
24. Hattori, T. and Fibiger, H.C. (1982): Brain Res. 238: 245-250.
25. Henderson, G., Hughes, J. and Kosterlitz, H.W. (1978): Nature 271: 677-679.
26. Hendry, S.H.C., Jones, E.G., and Emson, P.C. (1984): J. Neurosci. 4: 2497-2517.

27. Herkenham, M. and Pert, C.B. (1982): J. Neurosci. 2: 1129–1149.

28. Hunt, S.P. and Schmidt, J. (1978): Brain Res. 142: 152–159.

29. Jan, Y.N. and Jan, L.Y. (1982): J. Physiol., Lond. 327: 219–246.

30. Khachaturian, H., Lewis, M.E., Schäfer, M.K.-H. and Watson, S.J. (1985): Trends Neurosci. 8: 111–119.

31. Kuhar, M.J., Taylor, N., Wamsley, J.K., Hulme, E.C. and Birdsall, N.J.M. (1981): Brain Res. 216: 1–9.

32. Lentz, T.L. and Chester, J. (1977): J. Cell. Biol. 75: 258–267.

33. Lohl, H.H., Barse, D.A., Sampath-Khamma, S., Mar, J.B. and Way, E.L. (1976): Nature 264: 567–568.

34. Miller, R.J., Chang, K.-J., Leighton, J. and Cuatrecasas, P. (1978): Life Sci. 22: 379–388.

35. Mohler, H., Battersby, M.K. and Richards, J.G. (1980) Proc. Natl. Acad. Sci. USA 77: 1666–1670.

36. Murrin, L.C., Coyle, J.T. and Kuhar, M.J. (1980): Life Sci. 27: 1175–1183.

37. Parenti, M., Titrone, F., Olgiati, V.R. and Gropetti, A. (1983): Brain Res. 280: 317–322.

38. Penny, G.R., Wilson, C.J. and Kitai, S.T. (1984): Neuroscience Abstract 10: 514.

39. Pert, A. (1978): In: Characteristics and Function of Opioids, Van Ree and Terenius (Eds), Elsevier pp. 389–401.

40. Pert, C.B. and Snyder, S.H. (1973): Science 179: 1011–1014.

41. Pickel, V.M., Sumal, K.K., Beckley, S.C., Miller, R.J. and Reis, D.J. (1980): J. Comp. Neurol. 189: 721–740.

42. Pollard, H., Llorens-Cortes, C. and Schwartz, J.C. (1977): Nature 265: 745–747.

43. Quirion, R., Bowen, W.D., Herkenham, M. and Pert, C.B. (1982): Cell. and Mol. Pharmacol. 2: 333–346.

44. Quirion, R. and Weiss, A.S. (1983): Peptides 4: 445–449.

45. Reisine, T.D., Nagy, J.I., Beaumont, K., Fibiger, H.C. and Yamamura, H.I. (1979): Brain Res. 177: 241–252.

46. Roemer, D., Buescher, H.H., Hill, R.C., Pless, J., Bauer, W., Cardinaux, F., Closse, A., Hauser, D. and Huguenin, R. (1977): Nature 268: 547–549.

47. Roth, B.L., Laskouski, M.B. and Coscia, C.J. (1981): J. Biol. Chem. 256: 10117–10123.

48. Salpeter, M.M., McHenry, F.A. and Salpeter, E.E. (1978): J. Cell Biol 76: 127–145.

49. Schwartz, J.C., Pollard, H., Llorens, C., Malfroy, B., Gros, C., Prudelles, Ph. and Dray, F. (1978): In: Adv. Biochem. Psychopharmacol., E. Costa and M. Trabucchi (Eds), Raven Press, Vol. 18: pp. 245–264.

50. Simantov, R., Kuhar, M.J., Uhl, G.R. and Snyder, S.H. (1977): Proc. Natl. Acad. Sci. USA 74: 2167–2171.

51. Somogyi, P. Priestley, J.V., Cuello, A.C., Smith, A.D. and Takagi, H. (1982): J. Comp. Neurocytol. 11: 779–807.

52. Vincent, S.R., Hökfelt, T., Christensson, I. and Terenius, L. (1982): Neurosci. Lett. 33: 185–190.
53. Waksman, G., Hamel, E., Bouboutou, R., Besselièvre, R., Fournié-Zaluski, M.-C. and Roques, B.P. (1984): C.R. Acad. Sci. Paris 14: 613–615.
54. Waksman, G., Hamel, E., Fournié-Zaluski, M.-C. and Roques, B.P.: Proc. Natl. Acad. Sci. USA, in press.
55. Wamsley, J.K., Young, W.S. and Kuhar, M.J. (1980): Brain Res. 190: 153–174.
56. Watson, S.J., Akil, H., Sullivan, S. and Barchas, J.D. (1977): Life Sci. 21: 733–738.
57. Weber, E. and Barchas, J.D. (1983): Proc. Natl. Acad. Sci. USA 80: 1125–1129.
58. Weber, E., Evans, C.J. and Barchas, J.D. (1983): Trends Neurosci. 6: 333–336.
59. Williams, M.A. (1969): Adv. Opt. Electron Microsc. 3: 219–272.
60. Yang, H.Y., Hong, J.-S., and Costa, E. (1977): Neuropharmacology 16: 303–307.

Neurotransmitter Interactions in the Basal Ganglia, edited by M. Sandler et al.
Raven Press, New York © 1987.

THE ACTION OF DOPAMINE ON SYNAPTIC TRANSMISSION THROUGH THE STRIATUM

G.W. Arbuthnott, J.R. Brown[a], N.K. MacLeod[b],
R. Mitchell, A.K. Wright

MRC Brain Metabolism Unit, University Department of Pharmacology,
1 George Square, Edinburgh, EH8 9JZ.
a) J.R.B. is now at Glaxo Research Group, Ware, England.
b) N.K.M. is now in the Department of Physiology,
University of Edinburgh.

ABSTRACT

In experiments which include in vivo neurophysiological
investigations and studies of transmitter release in vitro we
have explored the relationship between the dopaminergic input to
the neostriatum of the rat and the cortical input to the same
structure. Although this was first described as 'presynaptic' it
seems from recent anatomical data that the morphological
substrate for the interaction between the putative amino-acid
input to striatal cells and dopamine containing terminals in not
an axo-axonic one. Reviewing the experimental results in the
light of the anatomical data suggests many areas of convergence
between ultrastructural and physiological data but there remain
interesting mismatches which may suggest other than synaptic
interactions between cortical and nigral terminals. On the other
hand the neurophysiological data support the anatomical
suggestion that it is upon the striatofugal cells that the
interactions take place.

INTRODUCTION

There seems little doubt that anatomically the most extensive
input to the neostriatum comes from the cerebral cortex. Yet it
is the loss of the dopamine (DA) containing input to the striatum
which results in the dramatic loss of motor function seen in
Parkinson's Disease. Hardly surprising then that this DA input
should receive most pharmacological attention. At least one of
its functions in the neostriatum may be to control the efficiency
of cortico-striatal synapses(2). An understanding of the
physiology and pharmacology of cortico-striatal transmission
might shed light on the mode of action of DA and perhaps suggest
possible alternative therapeutic strategies in diseases of the
basal ganglia.

Cortico-striatal synapses are located on the dendritic spines
of striatal neurones (9; 12) including the striato-nigral output

neurones(20). The degeneration of these synaptic boutons leads
to the reduction of a high affinity uptake system for acidic
amino-acids(5). Futhermore long term effects of cortical
ablation include the reduction of glutamate concentrations in the
ipsilateral neostriatum (6; 9).

The inference that the cortico-striatal pathway uses glutamate
as its transmitter which follows from the biochemical and
anatomical studies also receives support from neurophysiological
studies with extracellular and intracellular recording methods
which indicate that glutamate mimics the excitatory action of the
cortico-striate pathway (4;21;22).

Although the cells in striatum on which the cortical synapses
are made had been described as interneurones (12) it is now clear
that many of the cells of the striatum in fact project out from
the nucleus. We therefore tried to identify the cells we were
recording from in the striatum of the anaesthetised rat, by
stimulating the crus cerebri. Such stimulation would be expected
to act on striato-nigral axons (23;24) and the identification of
these cells by antidromic responses to stimulation provided a
means to recognise projection neurones.

These striato-nigral cells were invariably silent in
anaesthetised male rats (23) but could be induced to fire in
response to stimulation through a suitably placed cortical
electrode. The action of iontophoresed DA on these cells has
been described in detail (2) and the first part of this paper
deals with the reinterpretation of those results in the light of
the anatomical findings (7). We have included a report of our
attempts to analyse which of the amino-acid receptor groups seems
to be involved, which has not been previously published.

There are several reports that the release and uptake of
glutamate is changed by DA application in vitro (14;16;17).
Neurophysiological and neuropharmacological data concur in
suggesting a presynaptic site for the interaction of glutamate
and DA. The anatomical studies, however, not only do not provide
evidence for axo-axonic synapses but also suggest that the
neurophysiological data can be explained by a post synaptic
action localised to dendritic spines. Although clearly not all
the in vitro data are compatible with the neurophysiological
results there is no clear anatomical substrate for the action of
DA on glutamate release. On the other hand recent
neurophysiological data from Dr Garcia-Munoz laboratory (8)
suggests that the inverse relationship – of glutamate on DA is
also demonstrable. Earlier biochemical results suggest a similar
interaction (15) but the anatomical substrate is unclear.

The cortico-striato-nigral system

The experiments were performed on male albino Wistar rats
(250g body weight). The methods are described in detail in
earlier reports from this laboratory (2;23) and briefly consisted
of anaesthesia with halothane (2% in air during surgery 0.8%
thereafter maintained via an endotracheal tube). Stimulating
electrodes of the concentric type were used, one implanted in the

premotor cortex and another, angled at 46° to the vertical, in the crus cerebri.

Multibarrel iontophoresis electrodes with a fine recording electrode glued alongside (3) were advanced slowly through the head of the neostriatum, and cells responding to stimulation through the cortical electrode were identified. The units were also tested for a response to stimulation of the crus cerebri. Responses were considered antidromic if they showed:1.Constant latency of action potential at suprathreshold stimulation, 2.The ability to follow stimulation at high frequencies (> 100 Hz), 3. Collision of an antidromic action potential with an orthodromic action potential. Because of the silent nature of the output cells,the third criterion was usually met by evoking an orthodromic action potential with cortical stimulation or, if this was not possible, by applying glutamate to the cell by iontophoresis at very low ejection currents. Several cells which fulfilled the first two criteria but which did not fulfil the third, were discarded.

Iontophoresis of glutamate and aspartate also excited many of the cells and the influence of a variety of amino–acid antagonist drugs were tested first for differential effects on the response to these two agents and also against the excitatory action of cortical stimulation. Care was taken to compare the actions in the presence of antagonist with previous control responses. At least two amino–acid applications or post–stimulus histograms (at the same voltage stimulation) were recorded in order to compare with the response during application of antagonist. Cells whose response did not return to this control value were discarded.

The actions of DA and sulpiride were also studied. In the case of sulpiride the action was only clearly visible at cortical stimulation strengths close to threshold. Again at least two post–stimulus histograms at the same stimulus voltage were collected before and after the application of sulpiride.

The action potentials of all the cells were biphasic with a total duration of approximately 4msecs. Occasionally, a notch was seen on the rising phase of the action potential. At threshold antidromic stimulation this was revealed as an initial segment spike when the stimulus failed to invade the soma.

Most striatal neurones could be excited by electrical stimulation of the sensorimotor cortex (0.2–1.2mA; pulse width 0.2msec). The stimulation site was similar to that used by Schultz and Ungerstedt(18) and the stereotaxic co–ordinates are described in Tansey et al (23). The usual response to cortical stimulation was one spike per stimulus but in some cases 2 or 3 spikes per stimulus were observed from neurones which were normally silent.

At stimulus intensities lower than those required for 1 : 1 following, considerable variation in latency was observed. With increasing stimulus strength, there was a decrease both in the mean latency of the response and in the variation of the latency. Post stimulus histograms (PSTH) were constructed for 212 cells; the response latency ranged between 4 to 19msecs.

76 (31%) neurones from a population of 212 were found to be antidromically driven. The latency of the antidromic response varied between 4 and 16msecs, with a mean value of 9.4msecs. Sixty-eight cells (89.5%) were excited by cortical stimulation and 8 cells (10.5%) were completely unresponsive. Of these 8 cells, none failed to respond to iontophoretic glutamate. Table 1 summarises the pharmacological results on the likely amino acid involved in cortico-striatal transmission. Unfortunately, from these experiments it is hard to make any firm conclusion.

TABLE 1:

Antagonist Ejection current nA range (mean ± SEM)	Excitant No.of cells depressed/No.of cells tested (mean ± SE of depression)		
	GLUTAMATE	ASPARTATE	Cortical stimulation
[a]APV 35 – 50nA 41.0±1.8	7/11 (71.7±11.3)	9/9 (72.0±5.2)	8/10 (76.0 ± 5.2)
[a]γ DGG 25 – 60nA 41.0±2.8	9/9 (69.3±7.7)	7/7 (86.3±4.6)	7/7 (82.8±5.4)
[a]PDA 20 – 60nA 50.5±2.6	7/7 (44.0±11.2)	7/7 (66.6±3.2)	4/4 (90.5±3.5)
GDEE 60 – 130nA 89.0±6.8	6/10 (68.0±7.1)	2/5 (79.0±15.5)	1/8 (50)

a;(±) 2 amino-5-phosphonovalerate (APV); γ-D-glutamylglycine(γDGG); and cis-2,3-piperidine dicarboxylate (PDA) were generous gifts from Dr. J.C. Watkins.

The antagonists used have know specificities for the different types of amino-acid receptors(26). In table 1 they are arranged in descending order of activity on the so-called N-methyl-D-aspartate (NMDA) receptor. Unfortunately all of the antagonists have some activity at this site. L-glutamic acid diethyl ester (GDEE) is the least active. GDEE also antagonises glutamate more than aspartate and is the least active of the agents tried against the effects of cortical stimulation. It has been reported to block the effects of acetylcholine and so it is remotely possible that the poor antagonism of the cortical response may be a reflection of this added action.

On the other hand intracellular recordings in the cat suggest the opposite conclusion. NMDA preferring agonists have effects which are not mimicked by cortical stimulation and which are blocked by doses of antagonist which do not significantly reduce the response to cortical stimulation (10;11). There are both species and sampling differences in the two sets of experiments but it must be admitted that the results in the cat fit better with biochemical data which suggests that glutamate is the best candidate as transmitter.

Neurophysiology of DA action

FIG. 1.

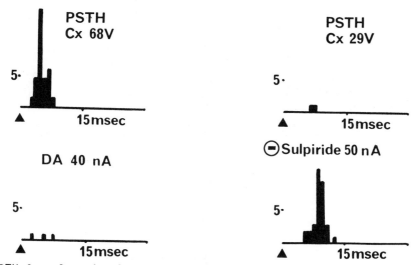

PSTH from 2 striatal cells in response to cortical stimulation are shown. On the left a brisk response to a high stimulus voltage is inhibited during the application of DA. On the right a small stimulus to cortex induces a smaller response which is increased during iontophoresis of -sulpiride at 50nM.

Dopamine iontophoresis during the collection of a PSTH always resulted in fewer responses being recorded in response to cortical stimulation (Fig. 1). In spite of biochemical evidence that the affinity for the DA binding sites associated with cortico-striatal axons is several times greater (19) we could never show this inhibitory action of DA at ejection currents which did not also reduce the response of the cell to applied glutamate. Fluphenazine (56-75 nA) antagonised the action of DA while sulpiride iontophoresis never did. Thinking that sulpiride might have a specific action which was being masked by the experimental design we attempted to study its action on cortico-striatal transmission itself. The iontophoretic application of (-) sulpiride clearly enhanced the effect of just suprathreshold cortical stimulation (Fig. 1). This effect was sterospecific and could be antagonised by DA — though only at doses which were themselves inhibitory on cortico–striatal transmission.

Biochemical action of sulpiride It seemed possible that the action in enhancing cortico–striatal transmission was a result of the action of sulpiride on D2 receptors. This conclusion was reinforced by the suggestion that the release of glutamate from striatal slices in vitro was inhibited by DA. Furthermore the D2 receptors were fewer in number in the striatum after decortication (19). We were encouraged to try to study the effect of sulpiride on glutamate release. There was already evidence that neuroleptics certainly did have actions on this preparation (14). Figure 2 shows the results. Sulpiride did not have an effect on resting glutamate release. It did inhibit the action of apomorphine on the glutamate overflow seen after K+ stimulation.

FIG.2.

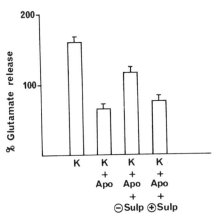

Peak glutamate response as a percent of basal (see 14) is shown for 4 different incubation conditions. The active isomer of sulpiride (–Sulp) significantly antagonises the reduction in potassium (K) stimulated release caused by apomorphine (APO).

Biochemistry and Neurophysiology do not always agree. In slices GABA had been shown to cause an increase of glutamate overflow (13). We therefore tested a few cells by iontophoresis of GABA during the neurophysiological experiments. In all cases GABA simply silenced the cells and made them inexcitable from the cortical stimulus. Of course this could have been the "cause" of the increased glutamate release via a local feedback, but since there was no convincing evidence for striato–cortical projections from dorsal striatum it was simpler to decide that it was not really possible to tie the biochemical and neurophysiological data too closely together.

<u>The effects of DA removal on the cortico-striato-nigral pathway</u>.
Specific lesions of the DA input to the striatum are possible
(25). We used animals so operated to try to see an effect on
the striatum which might relate the loss of DA to the action of
sulpiride. Two sets of results seem to support our idea that
the cortico-striato-nigral pathway was rendered hyperexcitable
by the lesion.

FIG. 3.

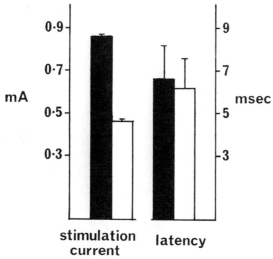

stimulation **latency**
current

Responses of striatal cells in 6-hydroxydopamine (6-OH-DA)
lesioned rats to cortical stimulation. The threshold
stimulation currents required to excite cells on the side of the
lesion (open column) were lower although the latency of response
from the cells was not different on the two sides.

Recordings were made from striatal cells and their threshold
to cortical stimulation noted. On the control side of the brain
(which still had an intact DA system) cells had very much higher
thresholds (Fig. 3). It seemed that sulpiride and the lack of
DA had similar effects on cortico-striatal transmission.
If the effect was relevant to the output cells on which we
had first observed it then we argued that it should also be
visible on the next cell in the chain. From a series of rats
with unilateral 6-OH-DA lesions in the nigro-striatal bundle
recordings were taken from the surviving cells in the substantia
nigra. Figure 4 illustrates the effect on the spontaneous
discharge pattern of nigro-thalamic cells identified, as we had
the striato-nigral ones, by constant latency and following
frequency as well as collision with orthodromic potentials.
Although the firing rates are lower on average the striking
change is in the number of really short intervals between action
potentials which was observed. Instead of the regular fast
discharge which normally characterises these cells they fire

with high frequency bursts (1).

FIG. 4.

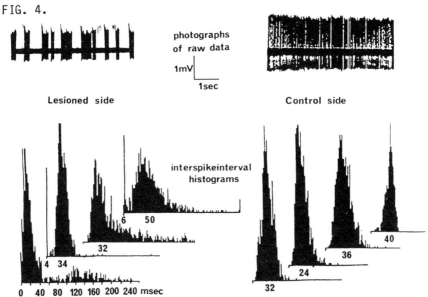

Oscillographic records and computer generated interspikeinterval
histograms from nigrothalamic neurones in 6-OH-DA lesioned
rats. On the side with the lesion most histograms are bimodal.
The numbers under the histograms show the modal intervals.

A reinterpretation in the light of fine structure
     The effects of DA, seemed to be equivalent to a presynaptic
inhibition of the cortical glutamate input to striatal cells.
Then Freund et al (7) published their study of the fine
structure of the striatal tyrosine hydroxylase containing fibres
in rat striatum.

FIG. 5. Synaptic arrangement of cortical and tyrosine
hydroxylase immunoreactive synapses on the dendritic spine of a
striatal neurone (after 7).

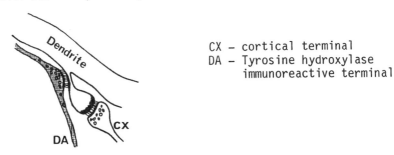

CX – cortical terminal
DA – Tyrosine hydroxylase
        immunoreactive terminal

The close association between assymetric synapses on the head of

dendritic spines and DA on the neck suggests a different
interpretation. Dopamine might have an effect whose specificity
on cortico-striatal synapses is the result of the anatomical
relationship between the synapses. How many of the observations
we have talked about so far are consonant with this
interpretation? The loss of D2 receptors after cortical lesions
can be explained as the result of the known loss of dendritic
spines which follows decortication(12). The specificity of
sulpiride for these receptors has allowed us to see its action.
Difficulties in access of iontophoresed DA to such a restricted
site might explain the absence of the 'order of magnitude
differences in potency' of DA at D_1 and D_2 receptors seen in
biochemical preparations. The D2 sites might well be more
sensitive but they were certainly less accessible. The
biochemical data still suggest an action of DA on the glutamate
terminals and that remains to be explained. Perhaps the close
association of the two endings allows for 'non-synaptic'
interactions. The glutamate terminals could be
pharmacologically sensitive to DA without there being any
synaptic interaction between terminals.

Before going too far with this heresy some interesting data
presented by Dr Garcia-Munoz at the "Dopamine 84" meeting in
Southampton (8) suggest that the close apposition of the two
terminals does allow physiological interactions. The
sensitivity of the terminals of DA neurones was tested by
stimulating in the striatum and recording the antidromic
threshold of the DA cells in the substantia nigra. Application
of excitotoxin or electrial stimulation (Fig.6) led to an
increase in the antidromic threshold which outlasted the
stimulation.

FIG. 6.

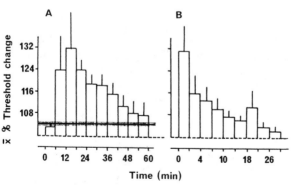

The mean change in threshold (± SEM; n = 24) after cortical
stimulation with (0.2µl: 6.8mM) Glutamate injection (A) or 1Hz
20sec trains of electrical pulses (B) at time zero is
illustrated. Threshold was the minimum electrical stimulation
required to activate the DA cell on 100% of non-collision trials.

The release of glutamate from cortical terminals had changed the electrical excitability of DA terminals. Perhaps these experiments are the electrophysiological reflection of the effect of cortical stimulation on DA release already reported in experiments with push pull cannulae in cats (15). Both results suggest that the triadic arrangement of the DA, glutamate and dendritic spine is capable of several levels of interaction. The changes in sensitivity of DA terminals could of course be the result of local ionic changes, but future experiments must test the specificity of the response and its pharmacology.

We are grateful to Drs. Garcia-Munoz and Chavez-Noriega for permission to use their unpublished results and to Celia Leitch for turning the last minute panic into a final manuscript.

References

1. Arbuthnott, G.W., MacLeod, N.K., and Ryman, A. (1984): J.Physiol.,358:43P.
2. Brown, J.R. and Arbuthnott, G.W. (1983): Neuroscience 10:349-355.
3. Brown, J.R., Mayer, M.L., and Arbuthnott, G.W. (1980): J. Neurosci.Methods 3:203-204.
4. Buchwald, N.A., Price, D.D., Vernon, L.and Hull, C.D. (1973): Exp. Neurol. 38:311-323.
5. Divac, I., Fonnum, F. and Storm-Mathiesen, J. (1977): Nature 266:377-378.
6. Fonnum, F., Storm-Mathiesen, J. and Divac, I. (1981): Neuroscience 6:863-873.
7. Freund, T.F.,, Powell, J.F. and Smith, A.D. (1984): Neuroscience 13:1189-1215.
8. Garcia-Munoz, M. and Chavez-Noriega, L. (1984): Presented at IUPHAR symposium Dopamine 84.
9. Hassler, R., Hang, P., Nitsch, C., Kim, J.S. and Paik, K. (1982): J. Neurochem. 38:1087-1098.
10. Herrling, P.L. (1985): Neuroscience 14: 417-426.
11. Herrling, P.L., Morris, R. and Salt, T.E. (1983): J. Physiol.(Lond) 339: 207-222
12. Kemp, J.M. and Powell, T.P.S. (1971): Phil. Trans. Roy. Soc. Lond. Ser. B. 262:383-401.
13. Mitchell, P.R. (1980): Europ. J. Pharmacol. 67:119-122.
14. Mitchell, P.R. and Doggett, N.S. (1980): Life Sciences 26:2073-2081.
15. Nieoullon, A., Cheramy, A., and Glowinski, J. (1978): Brain Res. 145:69-83.
16. Nieoullon, A., Kerkerian, L., and Dusticier, N. (1983): Exp. Br. Res. Suppl. 7: 54-65.
17. Rowlands, G.J. and Roberts, P.J. (1980): Europ. J. Pharmac. 62:241-242.
18. Schultz, W. and Ungerstedt, U. (1978): Brain Res. 142:357-362.
19. Schwartz, R., Creese, I., Coyle, J.T. and Snyder, S.H. (1978): Nature 271:766-768.

20. Somogyi, P., Bolam, J.P. and Smith, A.D. (1981) J. Comp.
     Neurol. 195:567–584.
21. Spencer, H.J. (1976): Brain Res. 102:91–101.
22. Stone, T.W. (1979): Brit. J. Pharmac. 67:545–551.
23. Tansey, E.M., Arbuthnott, G.W., Fink, G. and Whale, D.
     (1983): Neuroendocrinology 37:106–110.
24. Tulloch, I.F., Arbuthnott, G.W. and Wright, A.K. (1978):
     J. Anat. 127:425–441.
25. Ungerstedt, U. (1968): Europ. J. Pharmac. 5: 107–110.
26. Watkins, J.C. and Evans, R.H. (1981) Ann. Rev. Pharmacol.
     21:165–207.

Neurotransmitter Interactions in the Basal Ganglia, edited by M. Sandler et al.
Raven Press, New York © 1987.

FUNCTIONAL SIGNIFICANCE OF A DOUBLE

GABAERGIC INHIBITORY LINK IN THE STRIATO-NIGRO-FUGAL PATHWAYS

G. CHEVALIER and J.M. DENIAU

Laboratoire des Neurosciences de la vision
Université Pierre et Marie Curie, 4 Place Jussieu 75230 Paris
Cedex 05 France.

Neuropathological observations relating basal ganglia dysfunction to a wide variety of motor disorders have stimulated the study of the role played by this system with regard to the elaboration of movements. Since the functions of the basal ganglia are necessarily expressed through the structures which receive their influence, increasing interest has been paid to the analysis of the basal ganglia output pathways. There is now solid evidence that the internal segment of the globus pallidus (GPi or entopeduncular in rats and cats) and the pars reticulata of the substantia nigra (SNR) constitute major output systems of the basal ganglia, linking the striatum to various sensorimotor integrative centers of the diencephalon, mesencephalon and brain stem[19,25]. In rats for instance, SNR relays striatal outflow towards the intermediate strata of the superior colliculus (SC), some diffuse thalamic nuclei (ventral medial, central lateral/

medio-dorsal area, and parafascicular) and to the midbrain tegmentum[16].

In recent years, important progress has been made on the synaptic organization of the striato-nigro-fugal circuits which shed light on the way in which striatal activity might be translated into motor effects. In particular, attention has been focused on the GABAergic striato-nigro-collicular and striato-nigro-thalamic projection to the ventral medial nucleus (VM) since these pathways have been shown to be important for the expression of basal ganglia related motor syndromes such as: orofacial stereotypies, catalepsy and axiopostural deviations[13,28]. The purpose of the present paper is to give a brief survey of our present knowledge concerning the physiology of these GABAergic striatal output circuits.

A DOUBLE GABAERGIC INHIBITORY LINK IN THE STRIATO–NIGRO–COLLICULAR AND STRIATO–NIGRO–THALAMIC RELATIONSHIPS

It is today well established that the striato-nigro-collicular and striato-nigro-thalamic pathways include two successive GABAergic inhibitory links (fig 1). Indeed, the striato-nigral neurons which use GABA as a neurotransmitter[15,26,29] provide a very dense innervation of the SNR where they exert a potent inhibitory influence[1,14,27] on the nigrothalamic and nigrocollicular efferent neurons[8,9]. In turn these nigral efferent neurons are also GABAergic[2,12,24,31] and provide a powerful synaptic inhibitory effect on their thalamic[4,30] and collicular targets[3]. Considering such an organization we wanted to know how striatal activity might be expressed through these output circuits. An important clue was provided by the observation that in resting conditions (absence of active movements), SNR neurons maintain a sustained high frequency discharge (fig 1), while most striatal cells exhibit a very low level of firing. Thus it was suspected that the SNR exerts a tonic inhibitory control on its targets which might be transiently released as a result of a striatal discharge occuring for instance before the onset of goal directed movements. Through such disinhibitory mechanisms the striatal discharges would be translated into an increased excitability in tectal and thalamic circuits. To test such a hypothesis we ensured that SNR neurons really act on their tectal and thalamic targets by inhibiting them tonically. Next we determined whether striatal activity could trigger a discharge of tectal and thalamic cells by releasing them from the tonic nigral influence.

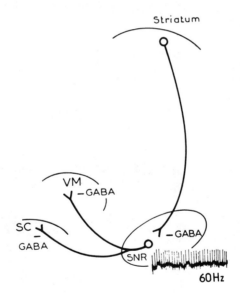

Figure 1 : Functional organization of striato-nigro-collicular and striato-nigro-thalamic relationships.
These striato-nigrofugal pathways are composed of double GABA-ergic inhibitory links. The inhibitory striatal influence is exerted on nigral neurons which are characterized by tonic back-ground activity. SC : Superior Colliculus ; SNR : Substantia nigra-pars reticulata ; VM : ventral medial thalamic nucleus.

The tonic inhibitory nigral control

If the inhibitory control of the SNR is tonic in nature, it would be expected that any change imposed on nigral background activity should be mirrored in an opposite manner in the excitability of tectal and thalamic cells. Conforming to this hypothesis we observed[6,11] that whereas a pause in nigral activity (produced by local application of GABA) is normally accompanied by a brisk and vigorous discharge in thalamic and tectal neurons, any increase in nigral firing rate (induced by intranigral application of bicuculline) silences them (fig 2).

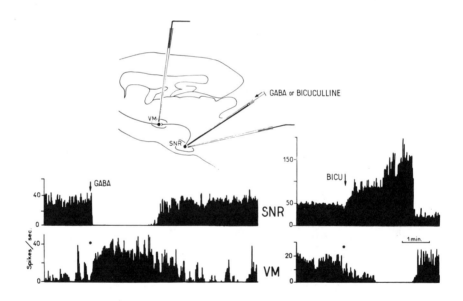

Figure 2 : *Demonstration that SNR exerts tonic inhibition on its targets.*
Single nigral and thalamic VM neurons were simultaneously recorded during pharmacological manipulations of nigral activity. Note that the nigral changes induced by local applications of either GABA or bicuculline are mirrored by opposite variations in thalamic background activity.

The disinhibitory striatal influence

Given the fact that SNR neurons really exert a tonic
inhibitory influence on their targets, it was of interest to
analyse how striatal discharges were translated through the
nigrothalamic and nigrotectal pathways. To achieve a selective
striatal stimulation we made use of local applications of
glutamate. By injecting this neuroexcitatory agent in volumes of
50 to 100 nl, we were able to induce sharp discharges of
striatal cells within a restricted portion of the nucleus (about
$1mm^3$).

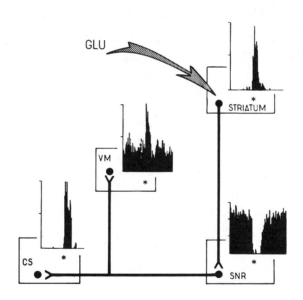

Figure 3 : Sequence of electrophysiological events induced
along the striato-nigro-thalamic and striato-nigro-collicular
system following activation of striatal neurons with glutamate
(GLU). The glutamate evoked discharge of striatal cells provo-
kes an inhibition of nigrofugal neurons which is secondarily
reflected in an excitation of thalamic and tectal cells via a
disinhibitory mechanism (* onset of glutamate injection in
striatum).

In response to such striatal activation, a majority (70 to 80%) of nigrothalamic and nigrotectal cells were silenced and, confirming our prediction, these striatally evoked nigral pauses were accompanied by a considerable increase in collicular and thalamic neuronal excitability[6,11](fig 3). We consider that these increases in collicular and thalamic excitability are actually generated through the double GABAergic disinhibitory striato-nigro-fugal pathways since:

-the use of a neuroexcitatory agent to activate striatal efferents ensures the specificity of the striatal stimulation. In particular, this procedure rules out the coactivation of striatal afferent fibers.

-the discharge of thalamic and collicular neurons is perfectly time locked to the striatally evoked silencing of nigral efferent neurons and it requires the integrity of the GABAergic neurotransmission within SNR   (fig 4).

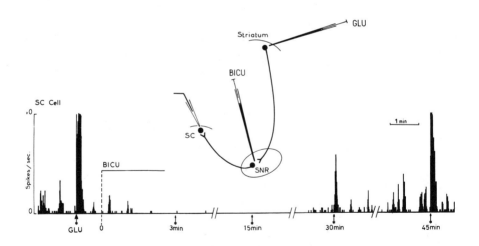

Figure 4 : Evidence for the involvement of a GABAergic intra-nigral link in the striatally evoked activation of tectal cells. Blockade of GABAergic neurotransmission in SNR by local appli-cation of bicuculline (BICU) prevents the SC cells from being fired from striatum (see trials 3 min. and 15 min. after BICU injection).

A DETAILED FUNCTIONAL ORGANIZATION IN THE
STRIATO-NIGRO-FUGAL PATHWAYS

In accordance with anatomical evidence that rat striato-nigro-fugal pathways present some topographic organization,[16,17] we observed that a given tectal or thalamic neuron can only be disinhibited from a restricted striatal locus[6,11]. Indeed, although the lateral region of striatum was particularly effective in activating thalamic and tectal neurons, a given cell was generally more sensitive to a particular locus within this area. This observation is probably due to the fact that nigro collicular and nigro thalamic cells receive their inhibitory influence from a restricted striatal region.

It is noteworthy that in addition to inhibitory effects, striatal stimulation can result in nigral excitation. As illustrated in fig 5, such opposite effects can be induced from the same striatal locus on closely located nigral efferent cells. Although the involvement of GABA in the striatally evoked nigral inhibition is clear, the origin of the striatal evoked excitations is still undetermined. These effects might result from the activation of striato-nigral peptidergic neurons[7]. However an alternative is to consider the intranigral interactions exerted by the inhibitory recurrent axonal network provided by each GABAergic reticulata neuron[10,20]. When a given set of nigral cells is inhibited by striatum, the surrounding neurons will presumably be excited through a disinhibitory process. Whatever their origin, these excitatory effects might allow a contrast enhancing process by which the disinhibitory action conveyed through the striato-nigro-collicular pathway could be focused on a particular set of collicular and thalamic cells.

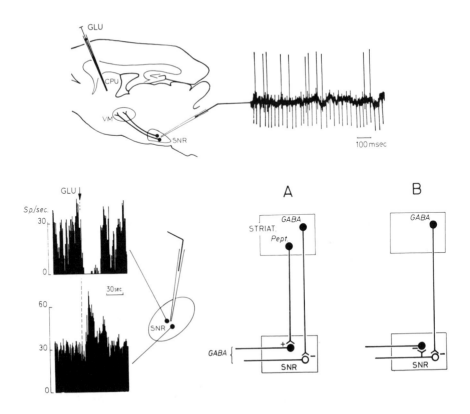

Figure 5 : Detailed functional organization within the striato-
nigrofugal pathways.
Two nigrothalamic neurons were concurrently recorded through
the same micropipette during an intrastriatal application of
glutamate (see experimental design on top of the figure).
Activities of the two cells could be easily differentiated
since the recorded potentials were of opposite sign. Their response to glutamate evoked striatal activation is shown in the
frequency histograms on the bottom left part of the figure.
Note that these two neighbouring nigral neurons responded in
an opposite way to the stimulation of a given striatal locus.
Diagrams A and B present two possible and non mutually exclusive origins for the excitatory effects evoked in nigral cells
induced from striatum. See text for further explanations.
CPU : Caudate/Putamen ; Pept : Peptidergic neurons ; STRIAT :
Striatum.

SOME INSIGHTS INTO THE FUNCTIONAL MEANING OF THE GABAERGIC LINKS
IN THE STRIATAL OUTPUT CIRCUITS.

To further our understanding on the physiological
significance of the GABAergic striato-nigro-fugal system, we
have identified some of the neuronal populations onto which
striatal information is channeled. From our present knowledge it
appears that through the nigrofugal pathways, striatal signals
will be predominantly addressed to centers involved in ocular,
cephalic and orofacial motricity. Indeed, at the level of the
SC, the striatum exerts its facilitatory influence on the
tectospinal/tectodiencephalic neuronal system[6] which projects
through its impressive axonal network to a number of structures
in diencephalon, rhombencephalon and spinal cord,[5,18] all
concerned with eye/head motricity. Moreover, at the level of
the ventral medial nucleus of the thalamus, striatal disinhibitory signals activate thalamocortical neurons[11]
innervating motor cortical areas devoted in particular to
orofacial and ocular movements. Recent studies in behaving
animals have revealed that the disinhibitory nigrofugal system
may be operational in the early stages of the initiation of
head/eye orienting movements. Indeed in cats[23] and monkeys[21,22]
it has been reported that the initiation of these movements is
generally accompanied by a clearcut arrest of the tonic nigral
activity.

Besides the SNR the GPi represents another key structure
involved in the transmission of striatal signals to premotor
centers. Interestingly, the striato-pallidofugal system is also
composed of two successive GABAergic inhibitory links.
Moreover, like nigrofugal cells, pallidofugal neurons are
tonically active. Thus it is very likely that the striato-
pallidofugal circuits also act via a disinhibitory process.

Consequently we propose that disinhibiton represents the basic process by which GABAergic striatal signals are converted into facilitatory influences on a wide spectrum of motor and premotor centers.

ACKNOWLEDGEMENTS

We are grateful to Dr S.J. Thorpe for reading through the text. This work was supported by INSERM grant (CRE 846006).

REFERENCES

1-Crossman,A.R., Walker,R.J.,and Woodruff,G.N. (1973): Brit.J. Pharmacol., 49: 696-698.

2-Chevalier,G., Thierry,A.M., Shibazaki,T., and Feger,J. (1981): Neurosci. Lett., 21: 67-70.

3-Chevalier,G., Deniau,J.M., Thierry,A.M., and Feger,J. (1981): Brain Res.,213: 253-263.

4-Chevalier,G., and Deniau,J.M. (1982): Exp. Brain Res., 48: 369-376.

5-Chevalier,G., and Deniau J.M. (1984): Neuroscience, 12: 427-439.

6-Chevalier,G., Vacher,S., Deniau,J.M., and Desban,M. (1985): Brain Res., 334: 215-226.

7-Cuello,A.C., Del Fiacco,M., Paxinos,G., Somogyi,P., and Priestley, J.V. (1981): J. Neural Transm., 51:83-96.

8-Deniau,J.M., Feger,J., and Le Guyader,C. (1976): Brain Res., 104: 152-156.

9-Deniau,J.M., Hammond,C., Riszk,A., and Feger,J. (1978): Exp. Brain Res., 32: 409-422.

10-Deniau,J.M., Kitai,S.T., Donoghue,J.P., and Grofova,I. (1982): Exp. Brain Res., 47: 105-113.

11-Deniau,J.M., and Chevalier,G. (1985): Brain Res., 334: 227-233.

12-Di Chiara,G., Porceddu,M.L., Morelli,M., Mulas,M.L., and Gessa,G.L. (1979): Brain Res., 176: 273-284.

13-Di Chiara, G., and Morelli, M. (1984): In Advances in Behavioral Biology: The Basal Ganglia, structure and function, edited by J.S. McKenzie, R.E. Kemm, and L.N. Wilcock, pp. 443-466. Plenum Press, New York and London.

14-Dray,A., Gonye,T.J, and Oakley,N.R., (1976): J. Physiol.,259: 825-849.

15-Fonnum, F., Gottesfeld, Z., and Grofova,I. (1978): Brain Res., 143: 125-138.

16-Gerfen,C.R., Staines,W.A., Arbuthnott,G.W., and Fibiger,H.C. (1982): J. Comp. Neurol., 207:283-303.

17-Gerfen,C.R. (1985): J. Comp. Neurol., 236: 454-476.

18-Grantyn,A., and Grantyn,R., (1982): Exp. Brain Res., 46: 243-256.

19-Graybiel,A.M., and Ragsdale,C.W. (1979). In: Development and chemical specificity of neurons, Prog. Brain Res. 51, edited by M. Cuenod, G.W Kreutzberg, and F.E. Bloom, pp. 239-283. Elsevier, Amsterdam.

20-Grofova,I., Deniau,J.M., and Kitai,S.T. (1982): J. Comp. Neurol., 208: 352-368.

21-Hikosaka,O., and Wurtz,R.H. (1983): J. Neurophysiol., 49: 1268-1284.

22-Hikosaka,O., and Wurtz,R.H. (1983): J. Neurophysiol., 49: 1285-1301.

23-Joseph,J.P, and Boussaoud,D. (1985): Exp. Brain Res., 57: 286-296.

24-Kilpatrick,I.C., Starr,M.S., Fletcher,A., James,T.A., and MacLeod,N.K. (1980): Exp. Brain Res., 40: 45-54.

25-Nauta,W.J.H., and Domesick V.B. (1984): In: Functions of the basal ganglia, Ciba Foundation Symposium 107, pp. 3-29. Pitman, London.

26-Oertel,W.H., Schmechel,D.E., Browstein,M.J., Tappaz,M.L., Ranson,D.H., and Kopin,J.J. (1981): J. Histochem. Cytochem.,29: 977-980.

27-Precht,W., and Yoshida,M. (1971): Brain Res.,32: 229-233.

28-Reavill,C., Jenner,P., and Marsden, C.D. (1984). In: Functions of the basal ganglia, Ciba Foundation Symposium 107, pp.164-176. Pitman, London.

29-Ribak,C.E., Vaughn,J.E., Saito,K., Barber,.R., and Roberts,E. (1980): Brain Res.,192: 413-420.

30-Ueki,A. (1983): Exp. Brain Res., 49: 116-124.

31-Vincent,S.R., Hattori,T., and McGeer,E.G. (1978): Brain Res., 151: 159-164.

Neurotransmitter Interactions in the Basal Ganglia, edited by M. Sandler et al. Raven Press, New York © 1987.

THE ROLE OF THE PRIMATE NIGROSTRIATAL DOPAMINE SYSTEM

IN THE INITIATION AND CONDUCTION OF BEHAVIORAL ACTS,

AS DERIVED FROM SINGLE CELL RECORDINGS

AND M P T P - INDUCED LESION EFFECTS

Wolfram Schultz

Institut de Physiologie, Université de Fribourg
1700 Fribourg, Switzerland

Through its involvement in Parkinsonism, the nigrostriatal dopamine (DA) system has classically been associated with motor functions. The additional non-motor deficits in this disease, which have recently become recognized (6), and the more general behavioral deficits in experimentally lesioned animals (8) point to a larger and more basic role of the DA system in behavioral acts. The present experiments were carried out in order to assess some of these functions electrophysiologically at the single cell level in unlesioned monkeys, and to compare these results to the deficits occurring in the same behavioral paradigm after a virtually complete lesion of the nigrostriatal DA system.

THE ACTIVITY OF DOPAMINE CELLS IN THE BEHAVING MONKEY

In continuation of an earlier study in which a different behavioral paradigm had been used (10), we recorded the electrical activity of single DA cells in the substantia nigra (SN) and its vicinity (areas A8, A9 and A10) in two Macaca fascicularis monkeys. Animals were seated in a primate chair and performed in a controlled paradigm involving the release of a holding key in response to the rapid opening of the door of a small food-containing box, with a following reaching movement of the hand into the box. A class of neurons was found in SN with electrophysiological characteristics, which were very similar to those of typical DA neurons in the rat (5). These neurons discharged spontaneously polyphasic, relatively long impulses (1.5 to 5.0 ms at 100 Hz high pass filtering) at low frequencies (0.1 to 8.0 imp/s), and were typically depressed in their activity by low doses of the DA agonist apomorphine (0.05-0.2 mg/kg s.c.). They clearly differed in these respects from pars reticulata cells, which discharged shorter impulses at higher frequencies and were not depressed by apomorphine.

Many DA cells responded to the behavioral trigger signal, i.e.
opening of the door of the food-containing box, with a latency
peak of about 100 ms (Fig. 1). This response occurred before the
following onset of movement but was time-locked to the behavioral
trigger. In addition to these responses, DA cells changed, mostly
increased, their activity moderately during the reaching movement, as also noted before (10). A few cells showed a relationship to the presence of the behavioral task, by changing their
activity tonically between onset of the task (closing of the door
by the experimenter) and its end (door opening with the following
movement). Some cells only showed changes at the very end of the
task during the time of reward-related mouth movements (see Table
1). These data show a direct relation of DA cell discharge
activity to the signal for immediately initiating a movement, and
to its execution.

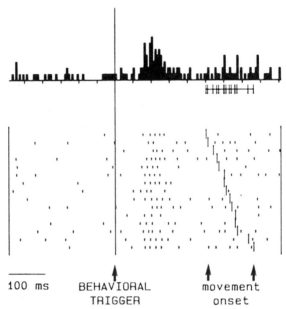

100 ms   BEHAVIORAL   movement
           TRIGGER   onset

FIG. 1. Extracellular discharge activity of a dopamine neuron in
monkey substantia nigra responding to the behavioral trigger
(door opening of a food-containing box) for arm movement. The
response is time-locked to the behavioral trigger (central solid
line) and not to the later occurring movement (small lines below
the histogram and in the right half of the dot display). Data are
shown in the form of a dot display in which each dot represents
the moment of a neuronal discharge, and each horizontal line of
dots represents one performance in the task. The sequence of
dotted lines is rearranged according to increasing intervals
between the behavioral trigger and movement onset (reaction
time). The peri-stimulus-time-histogram shown above is a sum of
the discharges in the dot display. Bin width is 5 ms.

TABLE 1. Relationships of monkey dopamine cell activity to stimulus-triggered movements

| | Activated | | Depressed | | Tested |
	N	%	N	%	N
Trigger stimulus	70	55	11	9	128
Movement execution	40	31	22	17	128
Reward phase	11	9	1	1	128
Task duration	4	5	1	1	77

N = number of cells

BEHAVIORAL DEFICITS AFTER LESIONS OF THE DOPAMINE SYSTEM

For this part, we have used the same behavioral paradigm employing arm movement in response to opening of the door of a food-containing box. We measured (i) electromyographic (EMG) reaction time to door opening in the extensor digitorum and the biceps muscles of the arm, (ii) reaction time (from door opening to key release), and (iii) movement time (from key release to box entry), before and after systemic administration of the DAergic neurotoxin 1-methyl-4-phenyl-1,2,3,6-tetrahydropyridine (MPTP) (1) in two monkeys.

Beginning at one or two days after MPTP administration, both animals showed a complete absence of spontaneous movements, a severe reduction and slowing of stimulus-triggered movements, paradoxical kinesia and hyperflexed posture. One of them in addition had activation tremor, rigidity, adipsia and aphagia. All symptoms ameliorated with L-Dopa treatment, particularly hypokinesia. Animals were quantitatively tested in the behavioral paradigm after they had partly recovered from the initial hypokinesia, and one animal under additional DA agonist treatment (bromocriptine together with L-Dopa and benserazide). All three movement-related parameters were consistently increased ($p<0.001$, Kolmogorov-Smirnov test) with several hundred to more than 2000 movements tested on each side in both monkeys: EMG reaction time by 80-87 %, reaction time by 44-102 %, movement time by 34-98 % (11). Histological and neurochemical assessments of the lesion showed a more than 95 % destruction of the nigrostriatal DA system in both animals, while sparing the mesocortical DA and other monoamine systems in one of them (11).

For illustrating the role of the DA system in stimulus-triggered behavioral acts, a comparison can now be made between the behavior-related DA cell activity in the unlesioned monkey ('positive image') and the behavioral deficits occurring after an MPTP-induced DA cell lesion ('negative image') in the same behavioral paradigm (Fig. 2). Dopamine cells are activated by the behavioral trigger (door opening) during the time of initiation of movement, and show a slow and moderate increase of discharge

rate during its execution (Fig. 2, above). Corresponding behavioral processes are impaired after an MPTP-induced DA depletion.
This is evidenced by prolonged reaction times for EMG and
movement, and by an increased movement time (Fig. 2, bottom).
However, the correspondence does not hold for self-triggered
movements. The strongest deficits in the akinetic MPTP-treated
monkey are found with initiation of spontaneous movements, but we
have never seen changes in normal DA cell activity during initiation of these movements.

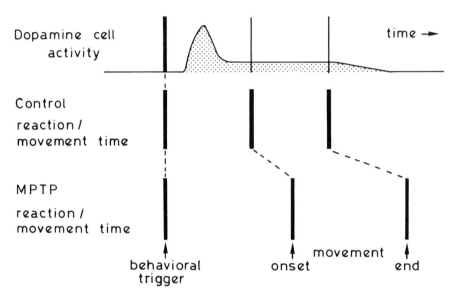

FIG. 2. A comparison between the behavioral relations of normal
dopamine neuron activity and the behavioral deficits occurring
after MPTP-induced dopamine cell lesions in the same behavioral
paradigm. The schematic representation of summed dopamine cell
activity shown above indicates a strong response to the behavioral trigger stimulus and a more moderate and slow activation
during execution of the movement. The behavioral deficits after
MPTP treatment comprise an increase in reaction time and in
movement time (lower part of the figure). Horizontal distances
between vertical bars indicate time intervals: reaction time
(from door opening as behavioral trigger to release of the
holding key as movement onset) and movement time (from movement
onset to entering the food box with the hand as end of movement).
It is interesting to note that dopamine neurons change their
activity during those parts of the behavioral paradigm in which
performance is impaired with a dopamine cell lesion.

THE FUNCTION OF THE DOPAMINE SYSTEM AS PART OF THE BASAL GANGLIA

The akinesia following lesions of the DA system in man and experimental animals consists of a general absence or reduction of all behavioral acts, rather than an impairment of certain details of motor performance. The activity of DA cells also shows a rather general relationship to the presence of behavioral activation, as expressed for example in movements (10). Therefore, the nigrostriatal DA system should not primarily be viewed under the aspects of motor control, but rather be associated with more general mechanisms of behavioral activation, which may for experimental reasons be divided into initiation and execution processes and studied with movements. In this function, the DA system influences postsynaptic structures of the basal ganglia which are closer linked to the details of the behavioral acts, i.e. the caudate nucleus and the putamen (Fig. 3). These two structures, respectively, are involved in sensory and movement initiation processes (7), and in the elaboration of certain movement parameters independent of the pattern of muscular activity (2). Movement-related neuronal information is conducted to the next synaptically linked structures, the pallidum and the pars reticulata of SN, where neuronal activity related to movements is found (3,9), and furtheron via ventral anterior thalamic nuclei to area 6 of cerebral cortex and to the primary motor cortex. Here, some neurons are engaged in the

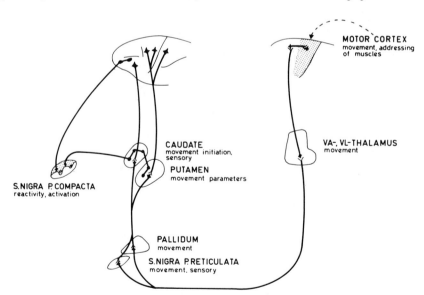

FIG. 3. A schematic representation of the flow of neuronal activity through the basal ganglia in relation to the initiation and execution of movements. For description see text.

direct addressing of motor units (4). Neuronal activity thus appears to become increasingly focussed onto the details of the motor act when progressing from the basal ganglia to the primary motor cortex, and parts of this information flow is controlled by the more basic behavioral activating mechanisms of the nigrostriatal DA system.

ACKNOWLEDGEMENTS

    This work is supported by the Swiss National Science Foundation (3.533-0.83) and the Sandoz Foundation. The neurochemical measurements were performed in collaboration with Drs. G. Jonsson, E. Sundström and I. Mefford at the Department of Histology, Karolinska Institutet, Stockholm, and supported by the Swedish Medical Research Council and a twinning grant from the European Science Foundation.

REFERENCES

1. Burns, R.S., Chiueh, C.C., Markey, S.P., Ebert, M.H. and Kopin, I.J. (1983): Proc. Natl. Acad. Sci. U.S.A. 80: 4546-4550.
2. Crutcher, M.D. and DeLong, M.R. (1984): Exp. Brain Res., 53:244-258.
3. DeLong, M.R. (1971): J. Neurophysiol., 34:414-427.
4. Fetz, E.E. and Cheney, P.D. (1980): J. Neurophysiol., 44:751-772.
5. Guyenet, P.G. and Aghajanian, G.K. (1978): Brain Res., 150:69-84.
6. Lees, A.J. and Smith, E. (1983): Brain, 106:257-270.
7. Rolls, E.T., Thorpe, S.J. and Maddison, S.P. (1983): Behav. Brain Res., 7:179-210.
8. Schultz, W. (1982): Progr. Neurobiol, 18:121-166.
9. Schultz, W., Aebischer, P. and Ruffieux, A. (1983): Exp. Brain Res. Suppl. 7:171-180.
10. Schultz, W., Ruffieux, A. and Aebischer, P. (1983): Exp. Brain Res., 51:377-387.
11. Schultz, W., Studer, A., Jonsson, G., Sundström, E. and Mefford, I. (1985): Neurosci. Letters 59: 225-232.

Neurotransmitter Interactions in the Basal Ganglia, edited by M. Sandler et al.
Raven Press, New York © 1987.

IN VIVO VOLTAMMETRY WITH CARBON FIBER ELECTRODES :

A TOOL FOR STUDYING DOPAMINERGIC NEURONS OF THE BASAL GANGLIA

F.G. Gonon, C.C. Mermet and F.M. Marcenac

INSERM U171 and CNRS LA 162, Hôpital Ste Eugénie, Pavillon 4H, 69230 ST GENIS LAVAL (FRANCE).

INTRODUCTION

Numerous electrochemical techniques combined with various kinds of electrodes have been used to monitor catecholamine derivatives in vivo (see ref. 30 for a review). An excellent introduction to these techniques has been recently published (27). In the present paper, we summarize some recent data on central dopaminergic neurons which were obtained by in vivo voltammetry used in combination with carbon fiber electrodes. There are no other reasons for the above restriction except the following one : the authors are thoroughly familiar with this special technique and feel more confident reporting on what they know well.

The active surface of the carbon fiber micro-electrodes developed by Wightman et al. (33) is the section of a carbon fiber which is 8 μm in diameter. On the other hand, that of the carbon fiber electrodes designed in our group is the whole surface of a carbon fiber 500 μm long and 12 μm in diameter (13). Despite these small sizes, it is obvious that these electrodes record the oxidation current of species which are present in the extracellular fluid. In this fluid, the oxidisable compounds found in the highest concentrations are ascorbic acid (AA, about 300 μM) and uric acid. Since the extracellular concentrations of catecholamine derivatives are much lower, (see below) special care must be taken to avoid overlap with the two acids mentioned above. Wightman's microelectrodes as well as our electrochemically

a) This work was supported by INSERM, CNRS and Université Claude Bernard (UER de Biologie Humaine).

treated carbon fiber electrodes, when both combined with pulse voltammetry allow separation of catechols from ascorbic or uric acid. In 1980, we demonstrated that the catechol present in the striatal extracellular space in the highest concentration is the direct dopamine (DA) metabolite : 3,4-dihydroxyphenylacetic acid (DOPAC)(10). The basal extracellular DA concentration appeared extremely low (in the 10-50 nM range)(11,15). These results have been confirmed by numerous studies performed with various electrochemical and perfusion techniques (17,28,34). The in vivo voltammetric monitoring of DOPAC with treated carbon fiber electrodes was used by several authors to further study the biochemical activity of dopaminergic neurons of the basal ganglia under various pharmacological and physiological conditions. These studies will be reviewed in the first part of this paper. In the second, we will discuss the approaches which have been developed by Wightman's group and in our laboratory, to monitor DA release.

I. IN VIVO MONITORING OF DOPAC

1. Significance of DOPAC variations :

When used in combination with differential pulse voltammetry, treated carbon fiber electrodes make the in vivo monitoring of the extracellular DOPAC level possible for several hours (up to 10) in several region of the basal ganglia of anaesthetized and conscious freely moving rats : substantia nigra pars compacta, ventral tegmental area (VTA), globus pallidus, caudate putamen, nucleus accumbens (ACC) and olfactory tubercle (OT)(2,11,22). According to post mortem studies, variations in DOPAC level are related to variations of catechol synthesis in dopaminergic neurons in physiological conditions and in most pharmacological ones except with drugs which inhibit monoamine oxidase or DA reuptake (32). Therefore, in vivo monitoring as well as post mortem assay of DOPAC levels may serve as a tool for studying variations in catechol synthesis. This assumption is supported by the fact that inhibition of catechol synthesis by alpha-methyl-para-tyrosine (AMPT) induced a decrease in DOPAC level (fig. 1). However, figure 1 shows that this decrease is more rapid for the DOPAC level recorded from VTA than from the striatum. This could be explained by the fact that, in terminal areas, high DA amounts are stored in vesicles. When the catechol synthesis is inhibited, DA is still released from the storage pool. Thus, the inhibition of DOPAC formation is delayed. On the other hand, in cell body areas DA is not stored in vesicles and this could explain why inhibition of catechol synthesis by AMPT or of monoamine oxidase by pargyline induced similar kinetics of decrease in the DOPAC level (fig. 1). This suggests that variations in the DOPAC level might be a better index of tyrosine hydroxylase activity in cell body areas than in the terminal fields.

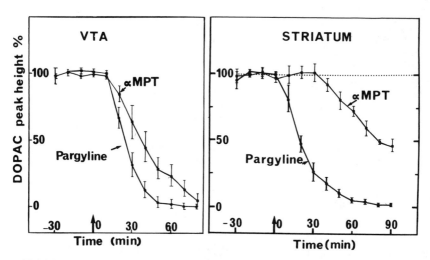

FIGURE 1 : Effect of AMPT (250 mg/kg, i.p.) and of pargyline (75 mg/kg, i.p.) on the DOPAC peak height recorded from the VTA and from the striatum. Recording from VTA was performed according to (2) except that the electrochemical techniques were as previously described (12). Data from the striatum are reproduced from (10). The vertical bars represent the mean ± S E.M. of n experiments expressed as previously (10).

2. Pharmacology of DOPAC variations :

Numerous drugs which are well known to act on biochemical activity of dopaminergic neurons (pargyline, amphetamine, reserpine, NSD 1015, AMPT, haloperidol, sulpiride, chloral hydrate, apomorphine), have been tested during in vivo monitoring of DOPAC in various brain areas (10,11,22). All the effects observed in these pharmacological experiments closely corresponded, in terms of amplitude and time course, to those of the same drugs on post mortem DOPAC levels. This excellent parallel confirms the identification of the catechol peak recorded with treated carbon fiber electrodes as being due to DOPAC.

Moreover, some of these studies provide new data concerning the pharmacology of DOPAC variations. Louilot et al. showed that sulpiride increases the extracellular DOPAC level in the olfactory tuberculum (OT) but not in the nucleus accumbens (ACC) of chloral hydrate anaesthetized rats. This higher sensitivity of the OT was also observed in conscious freely moving rats since 2 h after the injection of sulpiride (25 mg/kg) the DOPAC level reached 168 ±8 % of the control in the ACC and 210 ± 26 % in the OT (22).

It has been amply demonstrated that at a low dose, dopaminergic agonists decrease and antagonists enhance the discharge rate of dopaminergic cells by acting on autoreceptors located in substantia nigra and VTA. This prompted several authors to investigate in these regions the effect of these drugs on the biochemical activity of dopaminergic neurons. It was observed that haloperidol induced an increase in the post mortem DOPAC level in the substantia nigra and in the VTA (1,8). However, apomorphine was found unexpectedly ineffective on the same index (1,8). In order to further investigate this point, in the present study, we recorded the DOPAC peak from the VTA of anaesthetized rats and we observed that apomorphine (0.2 mg/kg, i.p.) induced a rapid decrease of this signal (fig. 2).

The role of these somatodendritic autoreceptors was studied using in vivo voltammetry by Maidment and Marsden. These authors recorded the DOPAC peak from the nucleus accumbens and observed that the amplitude of this signal was enhanced after a local haloperidol injection (2.5 µg/0.5 µl) in the VTA (25).

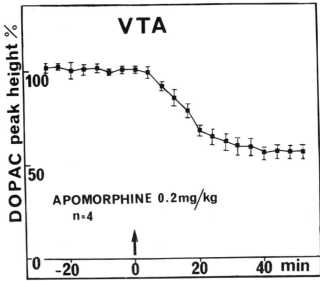

FIGURE 2 : Effect of apomorphine on the DOPAC peak height recorded from the VTA. The DOPAC signal was recorded every 2 min. in the same experimental conditions as in fig. 1.

3. DOPAC variations related to neurotransmitter interactions

Distinct dopaminergic neurons originating in the VTA innervate the ACC and the amygdala. However, from a functional point of view these neurons may be interdependent. Further, evidence in favor of this interdependence has been reported by Louilot et al. who recorded DOPAC in vivo in the ACC during local injections of tetrodotoxin and of dopaminergic drugs in the amygdala (23).

On the other hand, the interaction between serotoninergic and dopaminergic neurons was investigated with in vivo voltammetry by De Simoni et al. (5). The authors showed that electrical stimulation of the raphe dorsalis induces an increase in the striatal DOPAC level and that this effect is blocked by a serotoninergic antagonist (metergoline).

4. Behavioral studies

Louilot et al. (24) recorded the DOPAC level from the ACC of freely moving rats and observed that it was increased either by tail pinch (5 min.) or by a social interaction with a congenere (15 min.). In these conditions, the DOPAC signal reached 135 % of the control value and remained at this plateau at least 30 min. after the end of the stimulus. Thus, the authors suggested that this increased activity may correspond to a state of arousal. We agree with this opinion since we observed spontaneous variations in the DOPAC peak height recorded either from the ACC or from the OT (Gonon, preliminary unpublished results). The lowest values were recorded during the afternoon when rats were sleeping. At the beginning of the night when the light was turned off the rats became spontaneously active and this was always associated with a 25 to 35 % increase in the amplitude of the DOPAC peak.

II. IN VIVO MONITORING OF DA RELEASE

1. Methodological considerations

As pointed out in the introduction, due to its very low extracellular concentration, the in vivo electrochemical monitoring of DA is much more difficult than for DOPAC. In fact, up to now, in our opinion, no convincing evidence has been produced regarding the unequivocal in vivo monitoring of basal DA in drug free animals. In order to circumvent the difficulties two ways were feasible. The first one consisted of pharmacologically suppressing the voltammetric signal due to DOPAC and to use electrodes which cannot resolve DA from DOPAC but which are sensitive to DA in the nM range (12). The second approach was chosen by Wightman and coworkers who used untreated carbon fiber microelectrodes ; these electrodes exhibit a low sensitivity for DA but can separate DA from DOPAC. Therefore, these authors recorded the DA release which was evoked by electrical stimulation of the dopaminergic pathway.

2. DA release evoked by high frequency electrical stimulations

The micro-electrodes developed by Wightman et al. as well as our carbon fiber electrodes when they are not treated are able to unequivocally record DA in presence of physiological AA and DOPAC concentrations with a detection limit of 1 to 5 μM (6,15). Thus, they are not sensitive enough to record the basal extracellular DA concentration which is below 50 nM (see introduction). However,

they have been proved to be reliable for monitoring the DA release
evoked by electrical stimulations of the medial forebrain bundle
(MFB) provided that their frequency exceeds 30 Hz (6,20). In fact,
these stimulations induced an enormous increase in the
extracellular concentration. The highest effect (+ 65 μM) was
induced by a 60 Hz stimulation (20). This approach was used to
bring to the fore the low affinity, high capacity DA uptake by
extraneuronal elements (7,29). In another series of studies,
amphetamine which stimulates DA release, was found to attenuate the
effect of these high frequency stimulations (6,21). Although this
finding seems paradoxical at first glance, it is consistent with
in vitro studies (19) and give new insights into the two step
mechanism for the action of amphetamine on dopaminergic terminals
(21). Finally, Stamford et al. (31) investigated the role of AA on
the DA release evoked by electrical stimulations (50 Hz) and
showed that AA does not modulate this release.

3. Extracellular DA in terminal fields of pargyline treated rats

Although DA oxidizes on treated carbon fiber electrodes at
higher potential than DOPAC does (+ 85 mV instead of + 55 mV) and
although these electrodes are about 100 times more sensitive to
DA than to DOPAC (12), the extracellular DOPAC concentration is so
high that, in order to record a pure signal due to DA, we had to
suppress the DOPAC signal by pretreating the rats with a monoamine
oxidase inhibitor. When rats were treated with pargyline 3 h
before recording, treated carbon fiber electrodes used in
combination with differential normal pulse voltammetry (DNPV)
allowed us to record from the striatum and from the ACC a peak
appearing at + 85 mV. This peak was suppressed when the
dopaminergic terminals were selectively destroyed by a
6-hydroxydopamine injection in the substantia nigra. No peak was
recorded at + 85 mV when the tip of the electrode was implanted in
brain regions such as the frontal cortex, which are poorly
innervated by dopaminergic neurons. Finally, drugs which are known
to enhance DA extracellular concentrations (amphetamine,
methylphenidate, nomifensine, haloperidol) induced an increase in
the amplitude of this signal. Thus, the peak at + 85 mV which was
recorded from the striatum or from the ACC of pargyline treated
rats unequivocally corresponded to extracellular DA (15). By
calibrating in vitro, the electrodes after the in vivo recording,
the extracellular DA concentration was estimated to be 26 nM in
the striatum and 40 nM in the ACC. Imperato and Di Chiara showed
with trans-striatal dialysis that the DA release was enhanced by
pargyline (17). However, our estimate is lower than their by about
one half.

4. Extracellular DA and impulse flow

Electrolytical lesion of the medial forebrain bundle (MFB) as
well as apomorphine injection (50 μg/kg, s.c.) which strongly

inhibit the firing of DA neurons both induced an immediate 60 % decrease in the DA peak recorded from rats which were treated with pargyline and anaesthetized (15). This suggests that, in these conditions, only 40 % of the basal extracellular DA concentration corresponded to passive diffusion. However, this is probably an overestimate since, in these conditions, the discharge rate of DA neurons was probably lower than in normal ones. In fact, the mean discharge rate recorded from anaesthetized or paralysed animals seems lower than from chronic, freely moving rats (9) whereas pargyline does not modify this rate when injected in anaesthetized animals (B.S. Bunney, personal communication).

In recent studies, we investigated the effect of MFB electrical stimulations whose frequency never exceeded 20 Hz. This value corresponds to stimulations which mimic the highest spontaneous discharge rate of DA neurons since the shortest interspike interval recorded from chronic freely moving rats equals 51 ms (9). We found that these stimulations induced an immediate increase in the extracellular DA concentration and that this effect lasted as long as the stimulation did (at least up to 10 min.) (15,26). The amplitude of the effect depended on the frequency of the stimulation in an exponential manner (15). When a 20 Hz frequency stimulation was applied the DA concentration was increased from 26 nM to 146 nM (15). The amplitude of this effect is consistent with similar data obtained from trans-striatal dialysis (17). This suggests that, in normal conditions, the extracellular DA concentration remains below 200 nM.

Freeman et al. observed that DA neurons exhibit two firing patterns a single spike mode and a bursting activity. DA neurons can switch from one mode to the other and the bursting mode is often associated with an orientating response (9). Thus, it was suggested that changes in firing pattern may be an important method by which DA neurons modify DA release (16). In order to confirm this hypothesis we compared the effect of regularly spaced stimulations with bursted ones and we found that the latter were twice more potent than the former for the same number of pulses (14,15). Therefore, since a moderate increase in the firing rate of DA neurons is always associated with an increased burst firing (16), our finding suggests that the amplitude of variations in the DA release might be much higher than expected on the basis of changes in the mean discharge rate of DA neurons.

5. Effects of DA agonists and antagonists on extracellular DA

Tyrosine hydroxylase activity and discharge rate of DA neurons are both diminished by most DA agonists and enhanced by DA antagonists. Thus, the effect of apomorphine and of haloperidol on the impulse flow could be responsible, at least partly, for their effect on the extracellular DA concentration (see above). Moreover, numerous in vitro studies suggest that these drugs might act directly on DA release via an inhibitory autoreceptor located on DA terminals. We further investigated this mechanism by

recording in vivo the effect of these drugs on the DA release
which was evoked by low frequency electrical stimulations of the
MFB (14,15). Our results strengthen the validity of the
autoreceptor concept as an explanatory hypothesis for the effect
of dopaminergic drugs on DA release. However, the fact that the
amplitude of the DA release depends on the frequency of the
impulse flow in an exponential manner (15) does not suggest that,
at least in our conditions, extracellular DA per se actually
inhibits its own release.

6. Extracellular DA in VTA of pargyline treated rats

A dendritic DA release has been demonstrated in the pars
compacta of the substantia nigra and this release might control
the discharge rate of DA neurons through autoreceptors located on
dopaminergic dendrites (3). In accordance with this view, our
technique allowed us to record a DA peak from the VTA of pargyline
treated rats (fig. 3). The amplitude of this peak corresponded to
a DA concentration of 7-10 nM, and was increased by a subcutaneous
amphetamine injection. The figure 3 shows that haloperidol at
a low dose enhanced the extracellular DA level and this finding is
consistent with the above mentioned hypothesis concerning the
role of dendritic DA release.

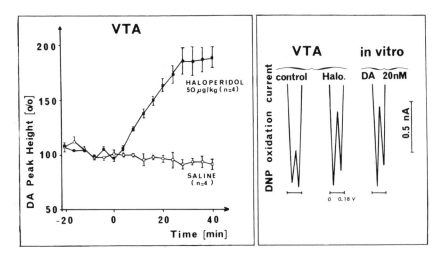

FIGURE 3 : Effect of haloperidol (50 µg/kg, i.p.) on the
extracellular DA concentration recorded from the VTA of
pargyline treated rats. The experimental conditions were as
previously described (15). The voltammograms shown in the
right part of the figure were recorded in vivo from the same
rat just before and 30 min. after the haloperidol injection.
Then, the same electrode was calibrated in vitro in a PBS
solution containing DA (20 nM).

7. Significance of extracellular DA

Since the extracellular space represents 15-20 % of the whole tissue volume (4), the synaptic cleft is a minute fraction of the whole extracellular space. Thus, relatively small amounts of DA released under the influence of the impulse flow could lead to a DA concentration into the synaptic cleft which might exceed the mean extracellular concentration by several orders of magnitude.

According to most estimates obtained with various techniques, in normal conditions, the extracellular DA concentration is below 200 nM. On the other hand, the DA concentration inside the DA terminals might be in the 1 mM range. Our guess is that the DA concentration which occurs in the synaptic cleft during the dopaminergic neurotransmission might be between these two extremes, namely in the 1 to 10 µM range. The extracellular DA which is actually monitored outside the synaptic cleft by voltammetric or perfusion techniques could reflect through a diffusion mechanism, and at a low level, the variations in DA concentration inside the synaptic cleft.

In a recent paper we suggested that, as regards dopaminergic neurotransmission, the extracellular space outside the synaptic cleft should be considered as an insulating space (15). In other words, this space might serve to restrict the dopaminergic transmission to the level of the synaptic contact and thus, to preserve the anatomical specificity of this chemical transmission. Recent morphological studies (see Bolam's chapter in this volume) demonstrate that most striatal dopaminergic nerve endings make symmetric synaptic contacts on the neck of dendritic spines of medium-sized spiny neurons. Thus, dopaminergic terminals were found to make highly specialized synapses and our hypothesis seems consistent with such findings.

REFERENCES

1. Beart, P.M., and Gundlach, A.L. (1980) : Br. J. Pharmac., 69 : 241-247.
2. Buda,M., Gonon, F., Cespuglio, R., Jouvet, M. and Pujol, J.F. (1981) : Eur. J. Pharmacol. 73 : 61-68.
3. Cheramy, A., Leviel, V., and Glowinski J. (1981) : Nature, 289 : 537-542.
4. Cragg, B. (1979) : Trends Neurosci. 2 : 159-161.
5. De Simoni, M.G., Giglio, R., Dal Toso, G., Kostowski, W., and Algeri, S. (1985) : Eur. J. Pharmacol., 110 : 289-290.
6. Ewing, A.G., Bigelow, J.C., and Wightman, R.M. (1983) : Science, 221 : 169-171.
7. Ewing, A.G., and Wightman R.M. (1984) : J. Neurochem., 43 : 570-577.
8. Fadda, F., Argiolas, A., Stefanini, E., and Gessa, G.L. (1977) : Life Sci., 21 : 411-418.
9. Freeman, A.S., Meltzer, L.T., and Bunney, B.S. (1985) : Life Sci., 36 : 1983-1994.

10. Gonon, F., Buda, M., Cespuglio, R., Jouvet, M., and Pujol, J.F. (1980) : Nature, 286 : 902-904.

11. Gonon, F., Buda, M., Cespuglio, R., Jouvet, M., and Pujol, J.F. (1981) : Brain Res., 223 : 69-80.

12. Gonon, F., Navarre, F., and Buda, M. (1984a) : Anal. Chem., 56 : 573-575.

13. Gonon, F., Buda, M., Pujol, J.F. (1984b) : In : Measurement of neurotransmitter release in vivo. edited by C.A. Marsden, John Wiley & Sons Ltd, Chichester.

14. Gonon, F. (1985) : In : Neurochemical Analysis of the conscious brain : voltammetry and push-pull perfusion. Ann. N.Y. Acad. Sci. : in press.

15. Gonon, F., and Buda, M.J. (1985) : Neuroscience, 14 : 765-774.

16. Grace, A.A., and Bunney, B.S. (1984) : J. Neurosci., 4 : 2877-2890.

17. Imperato, A., and Di Chiara, G. (1984) : J. Neurosci., 4 : 966-977.

19. Kamal, L.A., Arbilla, S., Galzin, A.M., and Langer, S.Z. (1983) : J. Pharmacol. Exp. Ther., 227 : 446-458.

20. Kuhr, W.G., Ewing, A.G., Caudill, W.L., and Wightman, R.M. (1984a) J. Neurochem., 43 : 560-569.

21. Kuhr, W.G., Ewing, A.G., Near, J.A., and Wightman, R.M. (1984b) : J. Pharmacol. Exp. Ther., 232 : 388-394.

22. Louilot, A., Buda, M., Gonon, F., Simon, H., Le Moal, M., and Pujol, J.F. (1985) : Neuroscience, 14 : 775-782.

23. Louilot, A., Simon, H., Taghzouti, K., and Le Moal, M. (1985): Brain Res., 346 : 141-145.

24. Louilot, A. , Le Moal, M. and Simon, H. (1985) : Neurosci. Let., Suppl. 22 : S557.

25. Maidment, N.T., and Marsden, C.A. (1985) : Brain Res., 338 : 317-325.

26. Marcenac, F. and Gonon, F. (1985) : Anal. Chem., 57 : 1778-1779

27. Marsden, C.A., Brazell, M.P., and Maidment, N.T. (1984) : In: Measurement of neurotransmitter release in vivo, edited by C.A. Marsden, pp 127-149. John Wiley & Sons, Chichester.

28. Sharp, T., Maidment, N.T., Brazell, M.P., and Zetterström, T. (1984) : Neuroscience, 12 : 1213-1221.

29. Stamford, J.A., Kruk, Z.L., Millar, J. and Wightman, R.M. (1984) : Neurosci. Let., 51 : 133-138.

30. Stamford, J.A. (1985) : Brain Res. Rev., 10 : 119-135.

31. Stamford, J.A., Kruk, Z.L., and Millar, J. (1985) : Neurosci. Let., 60 : 357-362.

32. Westerink, B.H.C. (1979) : In : "The neurobiology of dopamine" edited by A. Horn, J. Korf and B. Westerink pp 255-291, Academic Press, New York.

33. Wightman, R.M. (1981) : Anal. Chem., 53 : 1125A-1134A.

34. Zetterström, T., Sharp, T., Marsden, C.A. and Ungerstedt, U. (1983) : J. Neurochem. 41 : 1769-1773.

Neurotransmitter Interactions in the Basal Ganglia, edited by M. Sandler et al. Raven Press, New York © 1987.

DOPAMINE RECEPTOR MEDIATED INHIBITION
OF ^{3}H-ACETYLCHOLINE RELEASE

S. Arbilla, J.Z. Nowak and S.Z. Langer

Laboratoires d'Etudes et de Recherches Synthélabo (L.E.R.S.)
58, rue de la Glacière, 75013 Paris, France.

There is considerable evidence in favour of the existence of dopamine synapses on the dendrites of striatal cholinergic inter-neurons (21, 30, 39) which suggests a physiological interaction between dopaminergic and cholinergic transmission in the striatum (8, 16, 31). Biochemical studies of neurotransmitter turnover support the cholinergic link of dopamine-acetylcholine interactions. Accordingly, following the administration of the dopamine receptor agonist apomorphine, the release of acetylcholine is de-creased (9), the turnover of ^{14}C-acetylcholine is decreased (41) and acetylcholine levels are increased, presumably reflecting de-creased utilization of acetylcholine (15, 20, 32), and therefore suggesting the existence of a dopamine receptor which inhibits the activity of cholinergic neurons. In addition, the existence of a tonic dopaminergic influence on cholinergic neurons is sug-gested by the increase in acetylcholine turnover, which is pro-duced either by acute administration of dopamine receptor anta-gonists (6, 8, 15, 32, 40), or by the acute lesion of the dopam-inergic nigrostriatal axons (1).

THE RELEASE OF ^{3}H-ACETYLCHOLINE AS AN IN VITRO MODEL TO STUDY THE INFLUENCE OF DOPAMINE ON CHOLINERGIC NEUROTRANSMISSION

The study of the release of ^{3}H-acetylcholine formed from ^{3}H-choline in striatal slices in vitro offers a simple model for studying the modulation of cholinergic function by dopamine re-ceptors. Figure 1 shows a schematic representation of the in-teraction between dopamine and acetylcholine in the striatum. In experiments carried out in striatal slices, exposure to dopamine receptor agonists decreases the release of ^{3}H-acetylcholine evoked by either electrical stimulation or high potassium concen-trations (4, 10, 14, 22, 23, 35). In addition, an inhibitory ef-fect of released endogenous dopamine on depolarization-evoked release of ^{3}H-acetylcholine has also been reported. The magni-tude of this inhibitory effect is a function of the experimental conditions : the facilitation of the electrically-evoked release

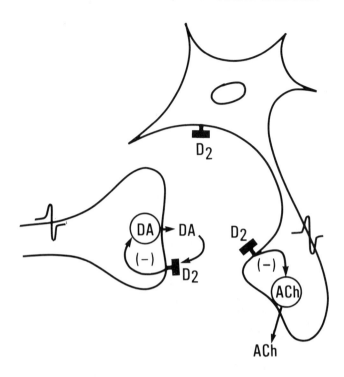

FIGURE 1 : Schematic representation of the interaction between
dopamine and acetylcholine in slices of the corpus striatum. Inhibitory D_2 dopamine autoreceptors involved in the regulation of
the release of dopamine are present in the dopaminergic nerve
terminal. In the cholinergic interneuron, inhibitory D_2 dopamine
receptors located in the nerve terminal or in the somatodendritic
area can modulate the release of acetylcholine. Dopamine receptors in the cholinergic interneuron can be activated pharmacologically or by endogenous dopamine under certain experimental conditions.

of ^{3}H-acetylcholine elicited by dopamine receptor antagonists is due to the blockade of the inhibitory action of endogenous dopamine, and it is observed only at high frequencies of nerve stimulation (10, 17). Thus, the activation of the dopamine receptors that inhibit the electrically-evoked release of ^{3}H-acetylcholine in rat striatal slices is a function of the synaptic concentration of released dopamine achieved in the synaptic cleft (10, 11, 17). The latter can be increased at high frequencies of stimulation, by inhibition of neuronal uptake of dopamine or through the displacement of newly synthetized dopamine by amphetamine (10, 11, 14, 17).

The release of dopamine in the striatum is modulated by inhibitory dopamine autoreceptors (26, 38) through a negative feedback mechanism. Accordingly, the removal of presynaptic receptor activation by dopamine receptor antagonists results in an enhancement of dopamine release (3, 10, 27, 38). Similarly to the situation that occurs at the level of dopamine receptors modulating ^{3}H-acetylcholine release, the facilitation of the electrically-evoked release of ^{3}H-dopamine by blockade of presynaptic inhibitory dopamine autoreceptors is also dependent on the frequency of nerve stimulation. Dopamine receptor antagonists facilitate the release of ^{3}H-dopamine at high frequencies of stimulation (3-10 Hz) more effectively than at lower frequencies such as 1 Hz (10, 24, 27).

PHARMACOLOGICAL CHARACTERISTICS OF THE DOPAMINE RECEPTORS THAT MODULATE THE RELEASE OF ^{3}H-ACETYLCHOLINE

As shown in Figure 2, the dopamine receptor involved in the inhibitory effect of apomorphine on the electrically-evoked release of ^{3}H-acetylcholine from rabbit caudate slices can be blocked by haloperidol and by the D_2 dopamine receptor antagonist sulpiride. Under the same conditions, the selective D_1 dopamine receptor antagonist SCH 23390 (25) is a weak blocking agent against the inhibitory action of apomorphine, which is in contrast to its potency in the nanomolar range to block dopamine-stimulated adenylate cyclase activity (25). The concentrations of haloperidol and sulpiride necessary to block the inhibitory effect of apomorphine on ^{3}H-acetylcholine release correspond to those that block the D_2 autoreceptor that modulates the release of ^{3}H-dopamine from the rabbit caudate (3). In support of these observations, the dopamine receptor involved in the inhibitory effect of amphetamine on ^{3}H-acetylcholine release is stereoselectively blocked by butaclamol and sulpiride, as well as by other dopamine receptor antagonists of different chemical series, with the exception of SCH 23390 (10). Conversely, with the use of selective dopamine receptor agonists of the D_1 and D_2 subtypes like SKF 38393 and LY 141865 respectively (37, 42), it was demonstrated that only the activation of D_2 dopamine receptors by LY 141865 influences cholinergic transmission in the rat striatum after its systemic administration (36). In addition, LY 141865

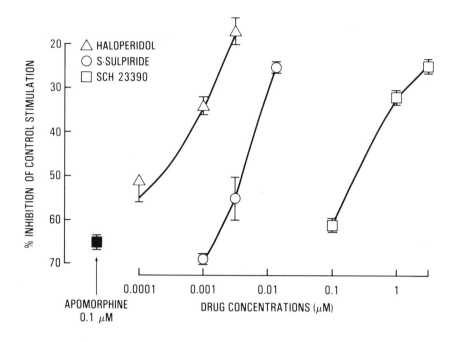

<u>FIGURE</u> <u>2</u> : Antagonism by different dopamine receptor blockers of the inhibition by apomorphine of the electrically-evoked release of ³H-acetylcholine. Rat striatal slices were labelled with ³H-choline and continuously perfused in Krebs medium. Two periods of electrical stimulation (1 Hz, 2 min), 44 min apart, were applied. The first period of stimulation corresponds to the control stimulation. Apomorphine 1 μM was added 20 min before the second period of stimulation. Dopamine receptor antagonists were present in the micromolar concentration indicated in the abscissa during both periods of stimulation. Ordinate : percent inhibition of the release of ³H-acetylcholine in the control stimulation. Shown are mean values ± S.E.M. of 3 - 5 experiments per group.

but not SKF 38393 inhibits the potassium-evoked release of ^{3}H-acetylcholine from striatal slices (36). Taken together, these results indicate that the activation of dopamine receptors of D_2 subtype results in the inhibition of cholinergic neurotransmission.

The pharmacological characteristics of dopamine receptors modulating ^{3}H-acetylcholine release in the striatum are similar to those of the dopamine autoreceptors that modulate ^{3}H-dopamine release (27, 29). Under similar experimental conditions, neither apomorphine (22, 28), nor molindone, sulpiride or metoclopramide (22) have been reported to distinguish between these two dopamine receptors. In spite of these pharmacological similarities, several pieces of evidence support the view that there are differences between dopamine autoreceptors and the postsynaptic receptors which modulate electrical activity of striatal neurons and mediate locomotion and stereotyped behaviour induced by dopamine receptor activation (28). Thus, it is not clear whether the dopamine receptor modulating ^{3}H-acetylcholine release represents a suitable model for the postsynaptic dopamine receptor that mediates the behavioural responses to dopamine agonists.

CHANGES IN SENSITIVITY OF RELEASE-MODULATING DOPAMINE RECEPTORS

The development of postsynaptic dopamine receptor supersensitivity after chronic treatment with neuroleptics is a well-established phenomenon (33). In addition, supersensitivity of presynaptic dopamine receptors after chronic neuroleptic administration has also been reported (7, 18, 19, 43). As shown in Figure 3, in rabbits treated for 28 days with haloperidol, there is a significant increase in the number of binding sites of ^{3}H-spiroperidol in the caudate nucleus when measured after 72 or 96 h of withdrawal from the drug. In slices of caudate nucleus from rabbits with 72 h withdrawal from haloperidol administration, it was observed that the presynaptic dopamine autoreceptors were supersensitive to the inhibitory effects of apomorphine (2, 34 ; Figure 4). In contrast, parallel experiments show that chronic treatment with haloperidol does not result in the development of supersensitivity to the inhibition by apomorphine of the electrically evoked release of ^{3}H-acetylcholine (Figure 4). In agreement with the lack of change of dopamine receptor sensitivity in the cholinergic interneuron after long term haloperidol administration, chemical denervation of the nigrostriatal dopaminergic neuron with 6-hydroxydopamine in rats does not result in changes in sensitivity to the inhibition by apomorphine of the electrically-evoked release of ^{3}H-acetylcholine (14). It should be pointed out that changes in sensitivity of transmitter release modulatory receptors can be demonstrated after chemical denervation of noradrenergic neurons with DSP4 at the level of inhibitory α_2-adrenoceptors modulating ^{3}H-5HT release from serotonergic nerve terminals in the rat hippocampus (12).

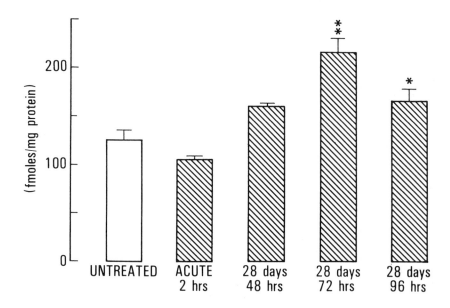

FIGURE 3 : Effects of repeated administration of haloperidol on ³H-spiroperidol binding to dopamine receptors in the caudate nucleus. Rabbits received one injection of haloperidol (1 mg/kg, s.c.), acutely or daily for 28 days, and were sacrificed 2, 48, 72 or 96 hs after the last injection (as indicated in the second line below each column). ³H-spiroperidol binding to dopamine receptors was determined as previously described (13). Columns represent the number of high affinity binding sites in fmol/mg protein at the concentration of 0.8 nM of ³H-spiroperidol. Values are mean ± S.E.M. from data obtained from at least 4 animals per group. ** $p < 0.001$ and * $P < 0.05$ when compared with the untreated group.

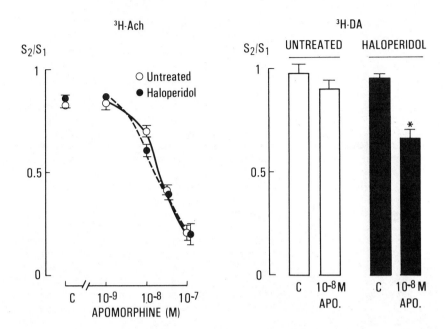

FIGURE 4 : Inhibition by apomorphine of the electrically-evoked release of ³H-dopamine and ³H-acetylcholine from rabbit caudate slices : influence of repeated haloperidol administration. Rabbits received one injection of haloperidol (1 mg/kg, s.c.) daily for 28 days and were sacrificed 48 h after the last injection. Values for the release of both transmitters are expressed in the ordinates as S_2/S_1 ratio. S_1 corresponds to the percentage of total tissue radioactivity released by the first period of stimulation, and S_2 to the second period obtained 50 min later. Apomorphine (APO) in the molar concentrations indicated was added 20 min before S_2. The values shown are the mean $\pm$ S.E.M. of 4 - 14 experiments per group, including at least 4 different rabbits. * $p < 0.01$ when compared with the control group in haloperidol treated animals. For experimental details, see References 26 and 34.

The inhibitory dopamine receptors modulating the release of ^{3}H-dopamine and ^{3}H-acetylcholine in the striatum do not develop the same adaptative changes following chronic blockade with haloperidol, suggesting differences in terms of their physiological involvement in the modulation of dopaminergic and cholinergic neurotransmission. The development of supersensitivity of the dopamine autoreceptors but not of the dopamine receptors in the cholinergic interneuron after haloperidol administration suggests that the dopamine autoreceptor is activated by released dopamine under physiological conditions of neurotransmission.

CONCLUDING REMARKS

The electrically-evoked release of ^{3}H-acetylcholine from striatal slices is modulated by inhibitory dopamine receptors of D2 subtype which are pharmacologically similar to the dopamine autoreceptors that modulate the release of ^{3}H-dopamine through a negative feed-back mechanism. The activation by endogenous dopamine of the dopamine receptors that inhibit the release of ^{3}H-acetylcholine is a function of the synaptic concentrations of dopamine, and it can be demonstrated by releasing dopamine at high frequencies of stimulation, by inhibition of the neuronal uptake of dopamine, or by displacement of dopamine with indirect amines like amphetamine.

Chronic administration of haloperidol produces supersensitivity to dopamine agonists at the level of dopamine autoreceptors modulating dopamine release, but fails to modify the sensitivity of dopamine receptors modulating ^{3}H-acetylcholine release in the caudate nucleus. It follows, therefore, that dopamine receptors modulating acetylcholine release in the caudate nucleus may not develop adaptative changes in sensitivity following chronic blockade with neuroleptics. It cannot be excluded, however, that dopamine receptors in the cholinergic interneuron can develop changes in sensitivity after repeated haloperidol administration, but the time course of the development of this phenomenon differs from that of the dopamine autoreceptor.

REFERENCES

1. Agid, Y., Guyenet, P., Glowinski, J., Beaujouan, J.C. and Javoy, F. (1975) J. Physiol. Lond. 312 : 397-334.
2. Arbilla, S., Bianchetti, G., Galzin, A.-M., Langer, S.Z., Morselli, P. and Nowak, J.Z. (1983) : Br. J. Pharmac. 78 : 16P.
3. Arbilla, S. and Langer, S.Z. (1981) : Eur. J. Pharmacol., 76 : 345-351.
4. Arbilla, S. and Langer, S.Z. (1984) : Naunyn-Schmiedeberg's Arch. Pharmacol., 327 : 6-13.
5. Arbilla, S., Nowak, J.Z. and Langer, S.Z. (1985) : Brain Res., 337 : 11-17.
6. Anden, N.E. (1972) : J. Pharm. Pharmac., 24 : 905-906.
7. Bannon, M.J., Bunney, E.B., Zigum, J.R., Skirboll, L.R. and Roth, R.H. (1980) : Naunyn-Schmiedeberg's Arch. Pharmacol., 312 : 161-165.
8. Bartholini, G. (1980) : Trends Pharmac. Science, 1 : 138-140.
9. Bartholini, G., Stadler, H. and Lloyd, K.G. (1975) : In : Cholinergic mechanisms, edited by P.G. Waser, pp. 411-418, Raven Press, New York.
10. Baud, P., Arbilla, S. and Langer, S.Z. (1985) : J. Neurochem., 44 : 331-337.
11. Baud, P., Arbilla, S., Cantrill, R.C., Scatton, B. and Langer, S.Z. (1985) : J. Pharmacol. Exp. Ther., 235 : 220-229.
12. Benkirane, S., Arbilla, S. and Langer, S.Z. (1985) : Eur. J. Pharmacol., 119 : 131-133.
13. Briley, M.S. and Langer, S.Z. (1978) : Eur. J. Pharmacol., 50 : 283-284.
14. Cantrill, R., Arbilla, S., Zivkovic, B. and Langer, S.Z. (1983) : Naunyn-Schmiedeberg's Arch. Pharmacol., 322 : 322-324.
15. Consolo, S., Ladinsky, H. and Bianchi, S. (1975) : Eur. J. Pharmac., 33 : 345-351.
16. Costa, E., Cheney, D.L., Mao, C.C. and Moroni, F. (1978) : Fedn Proc. Fedn Am. Socs Exp. Biol., 37 : 2408-2414.
17. Cubeddu, L.X. and Hoffmann, I.S. (1983) : J. Neurochem., 41 : 94-101.
18. Gallager, D.W., Pert, A. and Bunney, W.E.H. (1978) : Nature, 273 : 309-312.
19. Gianutsos, G., Hynes, M.D. and Lal, H. (1975) : Biochem. Pharmacol., 24 : 581-582.
20. Guyenet, P.G., Agid, Y., Javoy, F., Beaujouan, J.C., Rossier, J. and Glowinski, J. (1975) : Brain Res., 84 : 227-244.
21. Hattori, T., Singh, V.K., McGeer, E.G. and McGeer, P.L. (1976) : Brain Res., 102 : 164-173.
22. Helmreich, I., Reimann, W., Hertting, G. and Starke, K. (1982) : Neuroscience, 7 : 1559-1566.
23. Hertting, G., Zumstein, A., Jackisch, R., Hoffmann, I. and Starke, K. (1980) : Naunyn-Schmiedeberg's Arch. Pharmacol.,

315 : 111-117.

24. Hoffmann, I.S. and Cubeddu, L.X. (1982) : J. Neurochem., 39 : 585-588.

25. Iorio, C.L., Barnett, A., Leitz, F.H., Houser, V.P. and Korduba C.A. (1983) : J. Pharmacol. Exp. Ther., 226 : 462-468.

26. Kamal, L., Arbilla, S. and Langer, S.Z. (1981) : J. Pharmac. Exp. Ther., 216 : 592-598.

27. Lehmann, J. and Langer, S.Z. (1982) : Eur. J. Pharmacol., 77 : 85-86.

28. Lehmann, J. and Langer, S.Z. (1983) : Neuroscience 10 : 1105-1120.

29. Lehmann, J., Smith, R.V. and Langer, S.Z. (1983) : Eur. J. Pharmacol., 88 : 81-88.

30. Lloyd, K.G. (1978) : In : Essays in Neurochemistry and Neuropharmacology, edited by M.B.H. Youdim et al., pp. 129-207, Wiley, New York.

31. McGeer, P.L., Eccles, J.C. and McGeer, E.G. (1978) : In : Molecular Neurobiology of the Mammalian Brain, p. 452, Plenum Press, New York.

32. McGeer, P.L., Grewaal, D.S. and McGeer, E.G. (1974) : Brain Res., 80 : 211-217.

33. Muller, P. and Seeman, P. (1978) : Psychopharmacology, 60 : 1-11.

34. Nowak, J.Z., Arbilla, S., Galzin, A.M. and Langer, S.Z. (1983) : J. Pharmac. Exp. Ther., 226 : 558-564.

35. Scatton, B. (1982) : J. Pharmac. Exp. Ther., 220 : 197-202.

36. Scatton, B. (1982) : Life Sci., 31 : 2883-2890.

37. Setler, P.E., Saran, H.M., Zirkle, C.L. and Saunders, H.L. (1978) : Eur. J. Pharmacol., 50 : 419-430.

38. Starke, K., Reimann, W., Zumstein, A. and Hertting, G. (1978) : Naunyn-Schmiedeberg's Arch. Pharmacol., 305 : 27-36.

39. Tarsy, D. (1977) : In : Neurotransmitter function : basic and clinical aspects, edited by W.S. Fields, pp. 213-246, Stratton International, New York.

40. Trabucchi, M., Cheney, D.L., Racagni, G. and Costa, E. (1974) : Nature, 249 : 664-666.

41. Trabucchi, M., Cheney, D.L., Racagni, G. and Costa, E. (1975) : Brain Res., 85 : 130-134.

42. Tsuruta, K., Frey, E.A., Crewe, C.W., Cote, T.E., Eskay, R.L. and Kebabian, J.W. (1981) : Nature, 292 : 463-465.

43. Wheeler, S.C. and Roth, R.H. (1980) Naunyn-Schmiedeberg's Arch. Pharmacol., 312 : 151-159.

Neurotransmitter Interactions in the Basal Ganglia, edited by M. Sandler et al.
Raven Press, New York © 1987.

EXCITATORY AMINO ACID AND GABA INFLUENCE ON

RAT STRIATAL CHOLINERGIC TRANSMISSION

B. Scatton

Laboratoires d'Etudes et de Recherches Synthélabo
31 avenue Paul Vaillant Couturier
92220 Bagneux, FRANCE.

The striatum contains the highest levels of acetylcholine
(ACh), choline acetyltransferase, ACh esterase, high affinity
choline uptake activities and muscarinic receptor sites in the
central nervous system. The cholinergic activity in the
striatum is confined to intrinsic cholinergic neurons which
account for between 1 and 2% of the total neostriatal neuron
population (9,18). The cholinergic interneuron of the striatum
is relatively large (major axis in cross-section 25–30 μm) and
corresponds morphologically to the large, aspiny neurons of
Kemp and Powell (15) (dendritic spines are either very rare or
absent). These nerve cells appear to subserve an important
functional role in extrapyramidal motor function and have been
particularly implicated in the translation of alterations of
nigro-striatal dopaminergic activity into behavioral patterns
(see 20).

The relation of cholinergic neurons to striatal afferents
and other striatal neurons has been the subject of extensive
studies during the past decade.It is now well established that
striatal cholinergic neurons are controlled by the afferent
nigrostriatal dopaminergic (2,3,20) and raphé-striatal
serotonergic (8) pathways. The striatal dopamine-ACh balance
appears to be a major mechanism involved in the control of
extrapyramidal function.

Recent data obtained in our laboratory have suggested that
intra-striatal GABAergic neurons and cortico-striatal
glutamatergic pathways are also able to regulate striatal
cholinergic activity (19,28–33). The aim of the present chapter
is to review the available evidence for, and to analyze the
possible functional implications of, the excitatory amino-acid
and GABA influence on striatal cholinergic transmission.

121

EXCITATORY AMINO ACID INFLUENCE ON STRIATAL
CHOLINERGIC TRANSMISSION

Several lines of evidence suggest that striatal cholinergic interneurons receive a tonic excitatory input from the cerebral cortex which utilizes an excitatory amino acid, L-glutamate or L-aspartate, as its neurotransmitter. Thus, cortical ablation reduces high-affinity glutamate uptake (23) and concomitantly decreases ACh turnover (37) in the striatum. Similarly, systemic administration of the putative glutamate antagonist PK 26124 (2-amino-6-trifluoromethoxy-benzothiazole)(4,25) increases ACh levels (which reflects a decreased turnover of the transmitter) in the rat striatum (Fig. 1). Moreover, an input from the cerebral cortex onto the aspiny dendrites of neurons morphologically similar to the presumed striatal cholinergic interneurons is suggested by electron microscopical studies (11). Finally, the neurotoxic effect of kainate on cholinergic neurons (among others) in the striatum is abolished by prior lesioning of the cortico-striatal glutamate input and is restored in such lesioned animals by co-injection of glutamate (24). The fact that cortical ablation or injection of glutamate antagonists reduce striatal ACh turnover suggests that the cortical control of striatal cholinergic neurons is tonic in nature.

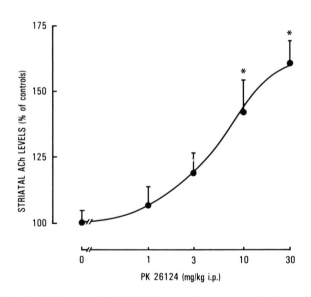

FIG. 1. Effect of PK 26124 on striatal ACh levels in the rat. *$p < 0.01$ vs controls.

Studies of physiological responses to a range of excitants and the discovery of preferential antagonists of amino acid-induced excitation in the vertebrate central nervous system has led to the classification of excitatory amino acid receptors into three subtypes, the N-methyl-D-aspartate (NMDA), the quisqualate and the kainate-preferring receptors (for review see 35,36). The NMDA receptor is preferentially activated by NMDA and antagonized selectively by a number of organic (phosphonate analogs of carboxylic acids) or inorganic (magnesium ions) agents. The second type of receptor is activated by quisqualate with L-glutamic acid diethyl ester (GDEE) and γ-D-glutamyl-aminomethylsulphonate (GAMS) as antagonists. The third receptor type is activated by kainate, insensitive to magnesium ions with no known specific antagonist. The naturally occurring amino acid neurotransmitters L-aspartate and L-glutamate seem to have mixed agonist actions at these proposed receptor sites, those for NMDA and quisqualate probably predominating in the excitation of central neurons by these amino acids when applied iontophoretically (35,36). Other endogenous compounds that are potent agonists at the NMDA type receptor include aspartate, quinolinic acid, L-cysteate, L-homocysteate and N-acetylaspartylglutamate.

We have recently attempted to characterize the pharmacological nature of the excitatory amino acid receptor(s) mediating the cortical excitatory influence on striatal cholinergic neurons by investigating the effects of specific excitatory amino acid receptor agonists and antagonists on the release of ^{3}H-ACh from slices of the rat corpus striatum (19,33). Because magnesium ions have been reported to antagonize the L-glutamate evoked neuronal depolarization (6), the release experiments were performed using magnesium-free medium.

Agonists of excitatory amino acid receptors caused an increase in striatal ^{3}H-ACh release. The relative order of potency was the following: NMDA > ($\pm$)ibotenate > N-methyl-DL-aspartate > L-glutamate > L-aspartate > quinolinic acid = kainate > quisqualate with EC_{50}'s ranging for 14 to 800 uM (Table 1).

This rank order of agonist potency in evoking ^{3}H-ACh release correlates quite well with the rank order determined electrophysiologically for NMDA-type receptors by Watkins (35,36) suggesting that the receptor which mediates the release of ^{3}H-ACh evoked by excitatory amino acid agonists is of the NMDA-type. This view is also supported by experiments performed with inorganic and organic antagonists of excitatory amino acids. Electrophysiological studies on spinal neurons have indicated that NMDA or L-aspartate but not kainate-induced responses are highly sensitive to magnesium ions (6,35). Similarly, we found that magnesium antagonizes (non

Table. 1 <u>Comparison of the potency of excitatory amino acid</u>
<u>receptor agonists to evoke, and of the potency of</u>
<u>excitatory amino acid receptor antagonists to</u>
<u>antagonize, NMDA (50 µM)-evoked, release of ^{3}H-ACh</u>
<u>from rat striatal slices (magnesium-free medium).</u>

Compound	EC_{50} (µM)	IC_{50} (µM)
Agonists		
NMDA	14	
NMDLA	50	
(+)Ibotenate	50	
L-Glutamate	200	
L-Aspartate	200	
Quinolinic acid	400	
Kainate	400	
Quisqualate	800	
Antagonists		(Against NMDA)
(−)APHept		40
(+)APPent		90
GDEE		> 1000
GAMS		> 1000

competitively) the release of striatal ^{3}H-ACh evoked by
N-methyl-DL-aspartate, (+)ibotenate and L-glutamate (EC_{50} 0.1
mM) but not by kainate (19,33).

As suggested by electrophysiological studies, excitatory
amino acid receptor subtypes exhibit a differential sensitivity
to blockade by specific organic antagonists. The two most
potent and selective antagonists of the NMDA-type receptor are
(−)2-amino-7-phosphonoheptanoate (−APHept) and (+)2-amino-5-
phosphonopentanoate (+ APPent) whereas, GDEE and GAMS act as
antagonists at quisqualate-type receptors (7,26). (−)APHept and
(+)APPent antagonized in a competitive manner the release of
^{3}H-ACh evoked by either NMDA or L-glutamate (Table 1)
(19,33). In contrast, the quisqualate receptor antagonists GDEE
and GAMS (up to 1 mM) failed to significantly affect the
responses to NMDA or L-glutamate (Table 1).

Taken together these experiments clearly indicate that the
receptor mediating the excitatory amino acid influence on
striatal cholinergic neurons resembles the NMDA-preferring
receptor as previously characterized electrophysiologically.
This contrasts with nigrostriatal dopaminergic neurons where
quisqualate-type receptors appear to mediate the excitatory
amino acid influence on dopamine release (27). A
quisqualate-type receptor regulating the release of L-aspartate
has also been identified in the rat hippocampus (21). It
appears therefore that the relative involvement of amino acid

receptor subtypes in the excitatory influence of amino acids on neuronal cells depends on the nature and/or regional localization of the target cells.

Since NMDA-type receptors mediate the excitatory amino acid influence on striatal cholinergic neurons, these receptors may play a part in transducing information received from the cerebral cortical afferents (which are thought to use L-glutamate or L-aspartate as neurotransmitter) to cholinergic cells. The question naturally arises as to the localization of those NMDA-type receptors modulating striatal cholinergic transmission. Since some excitatory amino acid receptors have been suggested to exist on nerve terminals (21,27), the excitatory amino acid receptor agonists may directly depolarize and initiate action potentials in cholinergic nerve terminals. However, although a direct depolarization of cholinergic nerve terminals by excitatory amino acid receptor agonists cannot be rigorously ruled out, the failure of N-methyl-DL-aspartate to evoke ^{3}H-ACh release from slices of hippocampus, interpeduncular nucleus and olfactory tubercle (19,32,33), where cholinergic afferents but not interneurons, are present, strongly argues against this possibility.

It is most likely that NMDA-type receptors are located on the dendrites of cholinergic neurons. Indeed, as stressed above there is anatomical evidence for an excitatory input onto the dendrites of striatal cholinergic interneurons (11). Moreover, tetrodotoxin (0.5 µM) abolishes the release of ^{3}H-ACh evoked by N-methyl-DL-aspartate and L-glutamate in magnesium-free medium (19,33). These data are consistent with the view that excitatory amino acid receptor agonists activate receptors located on cholinergic dendrites, causing depolarization and subsequent action potential propagation along the axons of the cholinergic interneurons to the terminals, where ^{3}H-ACh is released.

The involvement of NMDA-type receptors on cells other than cholinergic neurons which affect the cholinergic neurons via an unknown transmitter cannot, however, be totally ruled out. The cortico-striatal glutamatergic pathway is known to affect the release of striatal dopamine presumably via a direct presynaptic action at the dopaminergic nerve terminal (27, see also Chéramy et al, this symposium). Since dopaminergic neurons are involved in the transsynaptic regulation of striatal cholinergic neurons (2,3,20), dopaminergic neurons may also mediate the excitatory influence on striatal cholinergic neurons. However, the effects of NMDA on striatal ACh release are unlikely to be mediated via excitatory amino acid receptors on dopamine terminals, firstly because glutamate induced release of dopamine would be expected to reduce ACh release and secondly because chemical lesions of the nigrostriatal pathway do not affect the ability of NMDA or glutamate to increase striatal ACh release (32).

GABA INFLUENCE ON STRIATAL CHOLINERGIC TRANSMISSION

Ample evidence suggests that GABA exerts an inhibitory control over striatal cholinergic interneurons. Thus, systemic administration of GABA receptor agonists (e.g. progabide, muscimol) or indirectly acting GABA agonists (e.g. dipropylacetamide, γ-acetylenic GABA, nipecotic acid) 1) increases striatal ACh concentrations (Fig. 2A) (28-30), 2) reduces the formation of ^{14}C-ACh from 2-^{14}C pyruvate in striatal slices (30,31) 3) reduces the rate of utilization of striatal ACh (after hemicholinium-3 infusion into the striatum) in the rat (30,31). These data indicate a reduction of striatal ACh turnover by GABA agonists. As a consequence a GABA input may be involved in the regulation of the activity of striatal cholinergic cells.

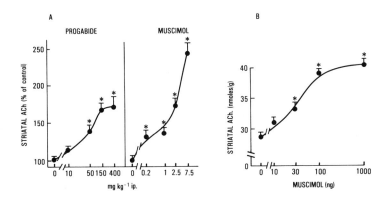

FIG. 2. Effect of systemic (A) or intrastriatal (B) injection of GABA receptor agonists on rat striatal ACh levels.

Rats were sacrificed 30 min after drug injection. Intra striatal infusion of muscimol was achieved by means of indwelling cannulae implanted 7 days before the experi- -ment. Results are means with SEM of data obtained on 10 rats per group.*p<0.05, **p<0.01 vs respective controls.

The inhibitory action of GABA on striatal cholinergic neurons does not seem to involve dopaminergic mechanisms. Thus, 1) as nigro-striatal dopaminergic neurons tonically inhibit striatal cholinergic cells (2,3,20), activation of GABAergic transmission, by reducing dopaminergic tone, would be expected to increase striatal ACh turnover 2) GABA mimetics cause a similar elevation of striatal ACh levels after chemical or surgical lesions of the nigro-striatal dopaminergic pathway or after pharmacological alteration of the activity of dopaminergic neurons (28,30,31).

The reduction of striatal cholinergic transmission by GABA appears to be mediated by intrastriatal mechanisms. Thus, intrastriatal infusion of GABA (750 ng) or muscimol (10-1000 ng) increases striatal ACh concentrations in the rat (Fig. 2B) (28,30,31). Moreover, intrastriatal infusion of the chloride channel blocker picrotoxin (0.25-1 µg) antagonizes the increase of striatal ACh levels elicited by a systemic injection of muscimol (5 mg/kg i.p.) (30,31). Finally, GABA reduces the potassium-evoked release of ^{3}H-ACh in perfused striatal slices of the rat (30,31).

Since the striatum contains a dense population of GABAergic interneurons (22), these neurons may directly impinge on cholinergic cells. However, the GABA influence on cholinergic neurons may also be exerted indirectly via a modulation of the activity of the cortico-striatal tract. Indeed, lesions of the cortico-striatal (glutamatergic) projections almost totally abolish the increase in striatal ACh concentrations elicited by systemic injection of GABA mimetics (29-32). Accordingly, the GABA-mediated inhibition of striatal ACh neurons may result from the stimulation of GABA receptors located on excitatory glutamatergic afferents to cholinergic interneurons: enhancement of GABAergic transmission would tune down excitation of striatal cholinergic neurons and thus lead to a decrease in ACh turnover. Another possible reason for the lack of effect of GABA on striatal ACh function after cortical ablation would be that such treatment results in transsynaptic degeneration of underlying cholinergic dendrites (see Bolam, this symposium)-presumably inducing loss of any receptors including those for GABA, normally localized on these dendrites.

In addition to the intrastriatal inhibitory GABA control, the cholinergic neurons also appear to be under an indirect facilitatory GABA influence mediated by the nigro-striatal dopaminergic neurons. Indeed, systemic administration of picrotoxin has been reported to increase striatal ACh levels, this effect being dependent on the integrity of the nigro-striatal dopaminergic pathway (13,17). Since dopaminergic neurons receive striato-nigral inhibitory GABA projections (10-12) and in turn tonically inhibit striatal cholinergic neurons (2,3), activation of GABAergic transmission is expected to reduce the inhibitory dopaminergic input on cholinergic cells, resulting in an increased ACh turnover. However, the reduced ACh turnover observed with GABA mimetics indicates that this indirect GABA facilitatory influence on striatal cholinergic neurons is of minor importance and is masked by the intrastriatal inhibitory GABA influence.

A possible explanation for the preponderance of the intrastriatal mechanism is that dopaminergic cells are in a state of tonic inhibition and thus show a low susceptibility to further inhibition by GABA whereas ACh-containing cells are inhibited to a lesser extent (possibly because they are under the excitatory influence of the cortico-striatal pathway) and are thus more sensitive to GABA agonists. Supportive evidence for this view is provided by the observation that the threshold dose of GABA mimetics for inhibiting cholinergic neurons is lower than that affecting the nigro-striatal dopaminergic pathway (1).

CONCLUDING REMARKS

The neuronal networks possibly involved in the transsynaptic regulation of striatal cholinergic transmission by excitatory amino acids and GABA are represented schematically in Fig. 3.

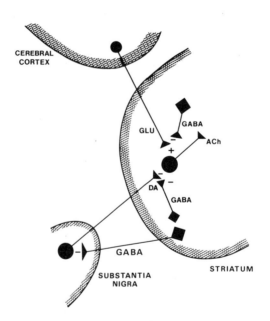

FIG. 3. <u>Schematic representation of the possible neuronal connections involved in the transsynaptic regulation of striatal cholinergic neurons by excitatory amino acids and GABA (GLU = glutamate, DA = dopamine)</u>

The present and previous studies provide evidence for an excitatory influence of excitatory amino acid pathways on cholinergic interneurons in the striatum, this excitatory influence being mediated by NMDA-type receptors. In the striatum, these receptors are located predominantly on the dendrites of cholinergic interneurons and may play a part in transducing excitatory amino acid neurotransmission carried by cortico-striatal afferents. GABA also modulates the activity of striatal cholinergic neurons 1) via an inhibitory action on the nigro-striatal dopaminergic neurons (facilitatory influence) and, in addition, a mechanism which is intrinsic to the striatum and mediated by GABA receptors on cholinergic cells and on the corticostriatal nerve terminals (inhibitory influence). The intrastriatal inhibitory GABA influence on ACh-containing cells predominates as compared to the dopamine-mediated facilitatory mechanisms.

The interactions between excitatory amino acid-, GABA- and ACh-containing neurons in the striatum may have important implications in the regulation of motor activities which are strongly associated with striatal cholinergic function (see Bartholini, this symposium for an extensive discussion). Intrastriatal application of NMDA has been shown to cause ipsiversive rotation (14) while intra-globus pallidus application of the compound induces locomotor hyperactivity and dyskinetic reactions (16). Therefore, excitatory amino acid receptor agonists and antagonists easily penetrating the blood brain barrier by acting on the glutamatergic inputs to the striatum and on the NMDA receptors that modulate striatal cholinergic neuron activity may prove useful in the treatment of neurological idiopathic or iatrogenic disorders (e.g. Parkinson's disease, tardive dyskinesias) associated with a relative dysfunction of the striatal cholinergic system.

On the other hand, while GABA mimetics (e.g. progabide or muscimol) given alone do not cause catalepsy or stereotyped behaviour, these agents at low doses potentiate apomorphine-, methylphenidate- and cocaine-induced stereotypies (1,34,38) and antagonize neuroleptic-induced catalepsy (1,38). These effects may be attributed to the inhibitory influence of these compounds on striatal cholinergic neurons ; in fact, at these low doses GABA mimetics decrease ACh turnover (see above). Furthermore, under these conditions, GABA agonists potentiate the apomorphine-induced increase in, and prevent the haloperidol-induced reduction of, striatal ACh levels (28,31).

On this basis, it is conceivable that GABA mimetics may be useful in the treatment of neurological disorders (e.g. Parkinson's disease) in which a relative exaggeration of cholinergic tone is known to be of aetiological importance. The available clinical results with progabide indeed indicate a positive effect of the compound on parkinsonian symptoms with a significant increase of the "on" time and a significant reduction of the severity of the "off" state (5).

REFERENCES

1. Bartholini, G., Scatton, B. and Zivkovic, B. (1980): In: Long-Term Effects of Neuroleptics, edited by F. Cattabeni, G. Racagni and F. Spano, pp. 207-214, Raven Press, New York.

2. Bartholini, G., Stadler, H., Gadea-Ciria, M. and Lloyd, K.G. (1975): In: Antipsychotic Drugs, Pharmacodynamics and Pharmacokinetics, edited by G. Sedvall, B. Uvnäs and Y. Zotterman, pp. 105-116, Pergamon Press, New York.

3. Bartholini, G. and Stadler, H. (1977): Neuropharmacology, 16:343-347.

4. Benavidès, J., Camelin, J.C., Uzan, A., Legrand, J.J., Gueremy, C. and Le Fur, G. (1985): Neuropharmacology, in press.

5. Bergmann, K.J., Limongi, J.C.P., Lowe, Y.H., Mendoza, M.R. and Yahr, M.D. (1984): Lancet 10:559.

6. Davies, J. and Watkins, J.C. (1977): Brain Res., 130:364-368

7. Davies, J. and Watkins, J.C. (1981): In: Glutamate as a Neurotransmitter, edited by G. Di Chiara and G.L. Gessa, pp. 275-284, Raven Press, New York.

8. Euvrard, C., Javoy, F., Herbet, A. and Glowinski, J. (1977): Eur. J. Pharmacol., 41:281-289.

9. Fibiger, H.C. (1982): Brain Res. Reviews 4:327-388.

10. Fonnum, F.I., Grofova, I., Rinvik, K., Storm-Mathisen, J. and Walberg, F. (1974): Brain Res., 71:77-87.

11. Hassler, R., Chung, J.W., Rinne, U. and Wagner, A. (1978): Exp. Brain Res., 31:67-80.

12. Hattori, T., Fibiger, H.C. and McGeer, P.L. (1975): J. Comp. Neurol., 162:487-504.

13. Javoy, F., Euvrard, C., Herbet, A. and Glowinski, J. (1977): Brain Res., 126:382-386.

14. Jenner, P., Marsden, C.D. and Taylor, R.J. (1981): Brit. J. Pharmacol., 72:570P.

15. Kemp, J. and Powell, T.P.S. (1971): Phil. Trans. Roy. Soc. Lond. B. 262:383-401.

16. Kerwin, R.W., Luscombe, G.P., Pycock, C.J. and Sverakova, K. (1980): Brit. J. Pharmacol., 68:174P.

17. Ladinsky, H., Consolo, S., Bianchi, S. and Jori, A. (1976): Brain Res., 108:351-361.

18. Lehmann, J. and Langer, S.Z. (1983): Neuroscience 10:1105-1120.

19. Lehmann, J. and Scatton, B. (1982): Brain Res., 252:77-89.

20. Lloyd, K.G. (1978): In: Essays in Neurochemistry and Neuropharmacology, edited by M.B.H. Youdim, W. Lovenberg, D.F. Sharman and J.R. Lagnado, pp. 129-207, Wiley, New York.

21. McBean, G.J. and Roberts, P.J. (1981): Nature 291:593-594.

22. McGeer, P.L. and McGeer, E.G. (1975): Brain Res., 91:331-335

23. McGeer, P.L., McGeer, E.G., Scherer, U. and Singh, K. (1977)
    : Brain Res., 128:369-373.
24. McGeer, E.G., McGeer, P.L. and Singh, K. (1978): Brain Res.,
    139:381-383.
25. Mizoule, J., Meldrum, B., Mazadier, M., Croucher, M., Ollat,
    C., Uzan, A., Legrand, J.J., Gueremy, C. and Le Fur, G.
    (1985): Neuropharmacology 24:767-773.
26. Perkins, M.N., Stone, T.W., Collins, J.F. and Curry, K.
    (1981): Neurosci. Lett., 23:333-336.
27. Roberts, P.J. and Anderson, S.D. (1979): J. Neurochem., 32:
    1539-1545.
28. Scatton, B. and Bartholini, G. (1980): Brain Res., 183:
    211-216.
29. Scatton, B. and Bartholini, G. (1980): Brain Res., 200:
    174-178.
30. Scatton, B. and Bartholini, G. (1980): Brain Res. Bull.,
    5, suppl. 2:223-229.
31. Scatton, B. and Bartholini, G. (1981): In: Cholinergic
    Mechanisms, edited by G. Pepeu and H. Ladinsky, pp.
    771-780, Plenum Press, New York.
32. Scatton, B. and Fage, D. (1985): In: Dynamics of Cholinergic
    Function, edited by I. Hanin et al., in press.
33. Scatton, B. and Lehmann, J. (1982): Nature 297:422-424.
34. Scheel-Krüger, J., Christensen, A.V. and Arnt, J. (1977):
    Life Sci., 22:75-84.
35. Watkins, J.C. (1981): In: Glutamate : Transmitter in the
    Central Nervous system, edited by P.J. Roberts, J. Storm-
    Mathisen and G.A. Johnston, pp. 1-24, John Wiley,
    Chichester.
36. Watkins, J.C., Davis, J., Evans, R.H., Francis, A.A. and
    Jones, A.W. (1981): In: Glutamate as a Neurotransmitter,
    edited by G.D. Di Chiara and G.L. Gessa, pp. 263-273,
    Raven Press, New York.
37. Wood, P.L., Moroni, F., Cheney, D.L. and Costa, E. (1979):
    Neurosci. Lett., 12:349-354.
38. Worms, P. and Lloyd, K.G. (1980): Naunyn-Schmiedeberg's
    Arch. Pharmacol., 311:179-184.

Neurotransmitter Interactions in the Basal Ganglia, edited by M. Sandler et al. Raven Press, New York © 1987.

ROLE OF CORTICOSTRIATAL GLUTAMATERGIC NEURONS IN
THE PRESYNAPTIC CONTROL OF DOPAMINE RELEASE

A. CHERAMY*, R. ROMO & J. GLOWINSKI

Chaire de Neuropharmacologie
INSERM U.114, Collège de France
11 place Marcelin Berthelot
75231 Paris cedex 05, France

In vitro studies performed on rat striatal slices
have shown that several transmitters which are contained in afferent or intrinsic fibers can influence
the spontaneous or evoked release of dopamine (DA)
from the nerve terminals of nigro-striatal DA neurons
(for review see 12). The effects of these transmitters
are mediated by receptors located either on DA nerve
terminals themselves or on other fibers or neurons
which could make axo-axonic contact or otherwise be in
close apposition with DA fibers. A direct effect is
indicated when the transmitter-evoked release of DA
still can be observed in the presence of tetrodotoxin
(TTX). This has been shown definitely for agonists
of L-glutamic acid, opiate and acetylcholine (ACh)
receptors (20,21,32). Binding studies in animals with
lesions of DA neurons also suggested the existence of
glutamatergic, muscarinic and enkephalin receptors on
these DA nerve terminals (6,7,17,24,26,36,41). Some of
the presynaptic regulations of DA release that have
been described in vitro also have been found in vivo
using halothane-anaesthetized cats implanted with
push-pull cannulae to measure the release of ^{3}H-DA
synthesized directly from ^{3}H-tyrosine (1,2,8,13,14,16,
19,43).

One important question that remains to be ans-
wered is how far presynaptic processes and nerve
impulse flow contribute to the control of DA transmission in the caudate nucleus in physiological condi-

---

*A.Chéramy is a research fellow of Rhône-Poulenc
Santé.

tions. During the last few years, we have obtained
evidence for the existence of a very potent facilitatory presynaptic regulation of DA release, mediated by
glutamatergic neurons originating in the cerebral
cortex which innervate the striatum massively. In
particular, the simultaneous recording of the activity
of DA cells and estimation of DA release from nerve
terminals has demonstrated that DA transmission in the
caudate nucleus is not dependent solely on the firing
rate of nigral DA cells.

Local effect of L-glutamic acid on DA release in the cat caudate nucleus

The effects of L-glutamic acid on ^{3}H-DA release
were investigated in cats implanted unilaterally with
a push-pull cannula in the caudate nucleus. Low
concentrations (10^{-8}M) of L-glutamic acid, added into
the superfusion medium stimulated markedly the release
of ^{3}H-DA synthesized from ^{3}H-tyrosine. This effect was
resistant to TTX ($5x10^{-7}$M) suggesting that it involved
glutamatergic receptors located directly on the DA
fibers. In addition, the stimulatory effect of L-
glutamic acid on ^{3}H-DA release was prevented when
tissues were superfused continuously with PK 26124, a
very potent antagonist of L-glutamic acid transmission. These results support in vitro data obtained on
rat striatal slices (20,37). Since complementary
ultrastructural observations have revealed that some
nerve terminals of cortical neurons are in close
contact with DA boutons (3), it can be concluded
tentatively that L-glutamic acid released from
terminals of cortical neurons exerts a direct presynaptic facilitatory influence on DA release.

Role of cortical glutamatergic neurons in the pre-synaptic control of DA release

In mammals, most, if not all, cortical areas
project to the striatum with a relatively precise
somatotopic organization (4,22,25,27,30,42). In the
cat, the sensori-motor cortex sends a massive
bilateral projection to the caudate nucleus (5). This
is not the case for other cortical areas, which
innervate predominantly the ipsilateral striatum only.
Although there is still some debate concerning the
identity of the transmitter contained in cortico-
striatal neurons, it is believed generally to be
L-glutamic acid, or a closely-related substance. In
fact, in the rat striatum, the levels of L-glutamic
acid and N-acetyl-aspartyl-glutamate, as well as the
high affinity uptake of L-glutamic acid, are decreased

markedly following a lesion of the prefrontal cortex (18,28,29). Excitatory responses produced by electrical stimulation of this cortical area are abolished in the presence of a L-glutamic acid antagonist (40).

In earlier investigations performed in cats implanted with two push-pull cannulae, we demonstrated that unilateral electrical stimulation of the pericruciate cortex produced a marked and sustained increase in DA release in both caudate nuclei, the effects being of similar amplitude (33). The contralateral effect was prevented by the sagittal section of the corpus callosum, which interrupted all crossing fibers, including those of cortical origin. These results, taken with the demonstration of a local stimulatory effect of L-glutamic acid on DA release, suggest that cortico-striatal glutamatergic neurons exert a presynaptic facilitatory influence on DA release mediated by glutamatergic receptors located on DA nerve terminals.

Several complementary observations indicate that presynaptic mechanisms play an important role in the *in vivo* control of DA transmission in the caudate nucleus of halothane-anaesthetized cats. 1) The blockade of sodium channels by TTX applied locally led to a 70% decrease in the spontaneous release of ^{3}H-DA indicating that a large part of the ^{3}H-transmitter recovered in superfusates is released in response to nerve impulse flow in the DA fibers themselves and in the striatal neurons that regulate them presynaptically. 2) A hemitransection made just in front of the substantia nigra, which interrupted all ascending fibers (including DA fibers), produced a decrease of only 30% in the spontaneous release of ^{3}H-DA suggesting that only about a half of the TTX-sensitive spontaneous release of ^{3}H-DA depends on impulse flow in DA neurons themselves. 3) Similarly, a 30% maximal decrease on the spontaneous release of ^{3}H-DA was observed during nigral (pars compacta) application of amphetamine (10^{-6}M), a treatment which increased markedly the dendritic release of DA and inhibited the firing of DA cells completely. 4) The spontaneous release of ^{3}H-DA was reduced by about 30% following a lesion (suction) of the ipsilateral pericruciate cortex. 5) Finally, the spontaneous release of ^{3}H-DA also was decreased by 30% when the caudate nucleus was superfused continuously with PK 26124, the potent L-glutamic acid antagonist. The latter two observations suggest that about half of the TTX-sensitive spontaneous ^{3}H-DA release is linked to impulse flow in cortico-striatal glutamatergic neurons, i.e. to

presynaptic facilitation of DA release by these
afferent fibers. These estimations however, should be
taken cautiously: it could be, for example, that both
hemitransection and local nigral application of
amphetamine may lead to an increased activity of
corticostriatal neurons. Changes in the activity of DA
cells, on the other hand, might occur following
destruction of the pericruciate cortex or the application of PK 26124 into the caudate nucleus. Finally,
other presynaptic facilitatory or inhibitory
influences also may contribute to the changes in DA
transmission observed in different experimental conditions.

Presynaptic facilitatory influence of the thalamo-cortico-striatal neuronal loop on DA release

Several processes contribute to the bilateral
regulation of DA transmission in the caudate nuclei.
Bilateral changes in DA release were seen not only
following unilateral electrical stimulation of the
pericruciate cortex (33), but also following unilateral pharmacological treatments made in the
substantia nigra (31,34,35), or in motor or intralaminar thalamic nuclei (15,38). Such changes also
were observed during electrical stimulation of either
the motor thalamic nuclei (10) or some nuclei of the
thalamic massa intermedia (11). Thus it seems that
nigro-thalamic neurons and efferent cells from motor
and/or intralaminar thalamic nuclei play an important
role in the interhemispheric regulation of DA transmission in both caudate nuclei (9,39). The mechanisms
involved in these bilateral changes of DA release seen
during unilateral modification of GABA transmission in
the motor thalamic nuclei (either VM or VL) have been
studied extensively. They have provided further
evidence for the contribution of presynaptic processes
in the control of DA release from the nerve terminals
of nigral DA cells.

In most experiments, cats were implanted with five
push-pull cannulae (one in each caudate nucleus, one
in each substantia nigra and one in the left VM or
VL). ^{3}H-DA released from nerve terminals and dendrites
was estimated ipsi- and contralaterally during and
after GABA application (10^{-5}M, 30 min) into the
thalamic motor nuclei. A marked and sustained stimulation of ^{3}H-DA release was observed in both caudate
nuclei and in the contralateral substantia nigra
whilst no modification of ^{3}H-DA release occurred in
the ipsilateral substantia nigra (15). Complementary
experiments suggested that the bilateral and symmetric

changes in DA transmission found in caudate nuclei were mediated by cortico-striatal glutamatergic fibers. 1) As had been observed previously in the case of unilateral electrical stimulation of the pericruciate cortex, the contralateral effect was prevented by sagittal section of the corpus callosum but not by sagittal section of the thalamic massa intermedia (39); 2) the ipsilateral effect still was observed following hemitransection, which interrupted all ascending fibers, including those of DA neurons; 3) the ipsilateral effect was abolished by local application of PK 26124, the L-glutamic acid antagonist which blocks the L-glutamic acid-evoked release of DA; 4) finally, changes of DA release in both caudate nuclei were no longer seen following ipsilateral lesion (local suction) of the pericruciate cortex.

Therefore, signals originating from thalamic motor nuclei (either VM or VL) due to the local application of 10^{-5} M GABA could reach the motor cortex and activate cortico-striatal glutamatergic fibers hence leading to the observed changes in DA release in the caudate nuclei.

Respective contributions of neuronal activity in DA cells and presynaptic mechanisms to the regulation of DA transmission

The next question was to determine the effect on the firing rate of DA cells of applying GABA into the thalamic motor nuclei. For this purpose, nigral DA cells were recorded extracellularly through microelectrodes introduced into the push-pull cannula. The activity of DA cells as well as the release of DA from dendrites and nerve terminals was estimated simultaneously.

The firing rate of DA cells was reduced markedly in both substantiae nigrae during and after unilateral application of GABA (10^{-5} M) into the thalamic motor nuclei (either VM or VL). Similar results were obtained when DA cells were recorded in animals not implanted with a push-pull cannula in the substantia nigra. Although we have no indication yet as to the identity of the inhibitory neuronal inputs responsible for the observed changes in the activity of DA cells, certain conclusions can be drawn from these combined electrophysiological and biochemical experiments. 1) DA release from nerve terminals can be enhanced despite inhibition of the activity of DA cells. This confirms the involvement of facilitatory presynaptic mechanisms. 2) Consequently, changes in DA transmission in the caudate nucleus cannot be deduced from measured changes in the firing rate of DA cells. 3) Changes in the activity of DA cells are not linked obligatorily to modifications of the dendritic release of DA. Indeed, although the increase in DA release in the contralateral substantia nigra induced by GABA (10^{-5}M) may have been responsible for the inhibition of DA cell firing, this was not the case in the ipsilateral side, since no significant modification of the dendritic release of DA was seen. This is not surprising, as inputs establishing synapses on the soma of DA neurons or on their proximal dendrites, may affect directly the firing rate of DA neurons. 4) In addition, complementary experiments indicated that distinct interhemispheric neuronal loops originating from thalamic motor nuclei were responsible for the GABA (10^{-5}M) -evoked release of DA in the contralateral caudate nucleus and substantia nigra. As discussed already, sagittal section of the corpus callosum prevented the contralateral effect in the caudate nucleus. The enhanced release of DA from dendrites, in contrast, was not abolished by this procedure. Conversely, sagittal section of the thalamic massa intermedia, which had no effect on ³H-DA release from nerve terminals did prevent the enhanced release of ³H-DA from dendrites (39).

Concluding remarks

In vivo studies performed in the cat have indicated that the cortico-striatal glutamatergic neurons exert a facilitatory influence on DA release in the caudate nucleus. This influence is linked to a presynaptic regulation mediated by glutamatergic receptors located on DA nerve terminals. This presynaptic regulation is bilateral and can be induced either by unilateral electrical stimulation of the pericruciate cortex or by unilateral application of GABA into the VM/VL thalamic nuclei. A thalamo-cortico-striatal neuronal loop is involved in this phenomenon, since lesion of the pericruciate cortex prevents the increase in ³H-DA release from nerve terminals seen following application of 10^{-5}M GABA into motor thalamic nuclei (either the VM or the VL). The latter treatment inhibited the firing rate of DA cells confirming that the increased release of ³H-DA in the caudate nucleus involved a presynaptic mechanism.

Previous observations indicate that facilitatory presynaptic regulation of DA release may or may not occur in the caudate nucleus, depending on the nature of the signals arriving from thalamic motor nuclei.

Signals originating in the substantia nigra and reaching thalamic motor nuclei (or intralaminar nuclei) via the nigro-thalamic neurons also may contribute to the regulation of the presynaptic facilitatory influence of cortico-striatal glutamatergic neurons on DA release. In fact, in earlier studies, bilateral symmetric changes in DA release had been observed in caudate nuclei following unilateral injections into one substantia nigra both of potassium (30 mM) and of drugs affecting GABAergic transmission (31,23). Experiments are therefore in progress to determine whether or not presynaptic regulation of DA release is important, either ipsi- or contralaterally in these situations. This study will provide a further paradigm in which to study the relative contributions of nerve activity in DA cells and of presynaptic regulatory processes in the control of DA transmission in the caudate nucleus.

Acknowledgements

This study was supported by grants from Rhône-Poulenc, DRET (83.084) INSERM and CNRS (ATP).

R. Romo is an IMSS fellow from Mexico. A. Chéramy is a Rhône-Poulenc research fellow.

We would like to acknowledge the valuable technical assistance of G. Godeheu and M. Saffroy.

References

1. BARTHOLINI, G., H. STADLER, M. GADEA-CIRIA & K.G. LLOYD (1976): Neuropharmacology, 15 : 515-519

2. BIGGIO, G., M. CASA, M.G. CORDA, F. VERNALONE & G.L. GESSA (1977): Life Sci. 21: 525-532

3. BOUYER, J.J., D.H. PARK, T.H. JOH & V.M. PICKEL (1984): Brain Res. 302: 267-275

4. CARMAN, J.B., W.M. COWAN & T.P.S. POWELL (1963): Brain 86: 525-562

5. CARMAN, J.B., W.M., COWAN, T.P.S. POWELL & K.E. WEBSTER (1965): J. Neurol. Neurosurg. Psychiat 28: 71-77

6. CAMPOCHIARO, P., R. SCHWARCZ & J.T. COYLE (1977): Brain Res. 136: 501-511

7. CHANG, R.S.L., V.T. TRAN & S.H. SNYDER (198): Brain Res. 190: 85-110

8. CHERAMY, A., A. NIEOULLON & J. GLOWINSKI (1978): Eur. J. Pharmacol. 48: 281-295

9. CHERAMY, A., V. LEVIEL, F. DAUDET, B. GUIBERT, M.F. CHESSELET & J. GLOWINSKI (1981): Neuroscience 6: 2657-2668

10. CHERAMY, A., M.F. CHESSELET, R. ROMO, V. LEVIEL & J. GLOWINSKI (1983): Neuroscience 8: 767-780

11. CHERAMY, A., R. ROMO, G. GODEHEU & J. GLOWINSKI (1974): Neuroscience Lett. 44: 193-198

12. CHESSELET, M.F. (1984): Neuroscience 6: 347-375

13. CHESSELET, M.F., A. CHERAMY, T.D. REISINE & J. GLOWINSKI (1981): Nature 291: 320-322

14. CHESSELET, M.F., A. CHERAMY, T.D. REISINE, C. LUBETZKI, M. DESBAN & J. GLOWINSKI (1983): Brain Res. 258: 229-242

15. CHESSELET, M.F., A. CHERAMY, R. ROMO, M. DESBAN & J. GLOWINSKI (1983): Exp. Brain Res. 51: 275-282

16. CHESSELET, M.F. & T.D. REISINE (1983): J. Neurosci. 3: 232-236

17. DEBELLEROCHE, J., Y. LUGUIANI & H.F. BRADFORD (1979): Neuroscience Lett. 11: 209-213

18. DIVAC, I., F. FONNUM & J. STORM-MATHISEN (1977): Nature 266: 377-378

19. GIORGUIEFF, M.F., M.L. LE FLOC'H, T.C. WESTFALL, J. GLOWINSKI & M.J. BESSON (1976): Brain Res. 106: 117-131

20. GIORGUIEFF, M.F., M.L. KEMEL & J. GLOWINSKI (1977): Neuroscience Lett. 6: 73-77

21. GIORGUIEFF, M.F., M.L. LE FLOC'H, J. GLOWINSKI & M.J. BESSON (1977): J. Pharmacol. Exp. Ther. 200: 535-544

22. GOLDMAN, P.S. & W.J.H. NAUTA (1977): J. Comp. Neurol. 171: 369-386

23. GREENFIELD, S., A. CHERAMY, V. LEVIEL & J. GLOWINSKI (1980): Nature 284: 355-357

24. GURWITZ, D., Y. KLOOS, Y. EGOZI & M. SOKOLOVSKI (1980): Life Sci. 26: 79-84

25. JONES, E.G., J.D. COULTER, H. BURTON & R. PORTER (1977): J. Comp. Neurol. 173: 53-80

26. KATO, G., S. CARSON, M.L. KEMEL, J. GLOWINSKI & M.F. GIORGUIEFF (1978): Life Sci. 22: 1607-1614

27. KEMP, J.M. & T.P.S. POWELL (1970): Brain 93: 525-546

28. KIM, J.S., R. HASSLER, P. HAUG & K.S. PAIK (1977), 132: 370-374

29. KOLLER, K.J. R. ZACZEK & J.T. COYLE (1984): J. Neurochem. 43: 1136-1142

30. KUNZLE, H. (1975): Brain Res. 88: 195-209

31. LEVIEL, V., A. CHERAMY, A. NIEOULLON & J. GLOWINSKI (1979): Brain Res. 175: 259-270

32. LUBETZKI, C., M.F. CHESSELET & J. GLOWINSKI (1982): J. Pharmacol. Exp. Ther. 222: 435-440

33. NIEOULLON, A., A. CHERAMY & J. GLOWINSKI (1978): Brain Res. 145: 69-83

34. NIEOULLON, A., A. CHERAMY & J. GLOWINSKI (1979): Science 198: 416-418

35. NIEOULLON A., A. CHERAMY, V. LEVIEL & J. GLOWINSKI (1979): Eur.J.Pharmacol. 53: 289-296

36. POLLARD, H., C. LLORENS & J.C. SCHWARTZ (1977): Nature 268: 745-747

37. ROBERTS, P.J. & N.A. SHARIF (1978): Brain Res. 157: 391-395

38. ROMO, R., A. CHERAMY, M. DESBAN, G. GODEHEU & J. GLOWINSKI (1983): Brain Res. Bull. 11: 671-680

39. ROMO, R., A. CHERAMY, G. GODEHEU & J. GLOWINSKI (1984): Brain Res. 308: 43-52

40. SPENCER, H.J. (1976): Brain Res. 102: 91-101

41. SUGA, M (1980): Life Sci. 27: 877-882

42. WEBSTER, K.E. (1965): J. Anat. (Lond.) 99: 329-337

43. WOOD, P.L. (1982): J. Pharmacol. Exp. Ther. 22: 674-679

Neurotransmitter Interactions in the Basal Ganglia, edited by M. Sandler et al. Raven Press, New York © 1987.

MODULATION BY DOPAMINE AND DOPAMINERGIC AGONISTS
OF ^{3}H-GABA RELEASED FROM STRIATAL AND
NIGRO-THALAMIC GABAERGIC NEURONES

M.J. Besson, J.A. Girault, U. Spampinato, M. Desban,
C. Gauchy, M.L. Kemel and J. Glowinski

Chaire de Neuropharmacologie - Collège de France
11, place M. Berthelot 75231 Paris cedex 05 - France

Nigrostriatal dopaminergic neurones play a strategic role in the functioning of the basal ganglia, witnessed by the massive sensorimotor deficits seen after their degeneration. These dopaminergic neurones have several well-characterized properties, among them that dopamine (DA) can be released not only from the nerve terminals which innervate massively the striatum, but also from the dense network of dendrites (6) in the substantia nigra pars reticulata (SNR) (3). Consequently, it was assumed that DA neurones might be involved in the control of the activity of both striatal neurones and nigral cells. Several electrophysiological studies have examined the action of DA on neuronal activity in both these structures, inhibitory and excitatory actions of DA or DA agonists have been described (2,5,23,34,39,45). Very little information is available concerning the action of DA on biochemically well-characterized neurones. The effect of DA agonists on cholinergic neurones of the striatum is one of the most clearly defined interactions: here, DA agonists acting on D2 receptors inhibit the release of acetylcholine (25). There is also some evidence for an interaction of DA with cortico-striatal fibres (40) containing glutamate (15) or related compounds (24) as their neurotransmitter, and with cholecystokinin fibres (27) present in the striatum. An inhibitory effect of DA on the release of GABA has also been obtained in this structure, although the paradoxical effects of DA antagonists in this system suggest a more complex action of the amine (7,43).

Since the measurement of the release of a neurotransmitter is an appropriate approach to the study of interactions between biochemically defined neurones, we have examined the effects produced by DA or DA agonists on striatal and nigral GABA neurones by measuring the release of ^{3}H-GABA in the striatum or in the thalamic terminal field of nigral efferent neurones. The release of ³H-GABA was measured in the rat striatum and in motor or intralaminar nuclei in the cat thalamus. Halothane anaesthetized animals were used, in which the structure of interest was superfused continuously, through a push pull cannula with a physiological medium containing ³H-glutamine as a precursor of ³H-GABA. The release of ³H-GABA was measured in serial 10 minute fractions.

EFFECTS OF DA AGONISTS AND ANTAGONISTS ON ³H-GABA RELEASE IN THE RAT STRIATUM

In the striatum, at least two distinct neuronal populations contain GABA as a neurotransmitter, interneurones (4) (medium-sized neurones with aspiny dendrites) and efferent neurones (medium-sized spiny neurones) sending projections to the pallidum and the substantia nigra (14,22,24) and giving rise to numerous recurrent collaterals into the striatum (32). These two neuronal populations can both contribute to the amount of the released ³H-GABA detected in superfusates collected in vivo from the rat striatum. The neuronal origin of ³H-GABA released is attested to by the fact that depolarization of the cells induced by addition of K^+ ions (30 mM-4 min) to the superfusion medium increased the release of ³H-GABA (+500%). This increased release was almost entirely Ca^{++} - dependent: a reduction of about 90% of the K^+-evoked release was observed following removal of Ca^{++} from the superfusion medium. This indicates that the contribution of glial cells to this release process is minor, since only the K^+-evoked release of GABA from the glial compartment is Ca^{++}-independent (37). However, the release of ³H-GABA seems only partly to be dependent on nerve impulse flow. In fact, addition of tetrodotoxin (TTX- a toxin acting on the fast Na^+ channels) to the superfusion medium produced a partial reduction (-25%) of the resting release of ³H-GABA. The mechanisms underlying the TTX resistant release are unknown, but it can be postulated that, as in other systems, a carrier-mediated transport contributes to the TTX resistant release (47). It should also be noted that a slight decrease in the release of endogenous GABA has been observed following TTX application in other in vivo studies (44).

Opposing Effects of D1 and D2 Agonists on the Release of ³H-GABA in the Dorsal Part of the Striatum

In the striatum, two well defined DA receptor subtypes have been described : the D1 and D2 receptors, whose stimulation leads to activation and inhibition of adenylate cyclase respectively (21,46). To investigate the possible control exerted by DA neurones on striatal GABAergic neurones, the effects of selective D1 or D2 agonists and antagonists on the release of ³H-GABA were investigated (see Table 1).

Addition of ADTN, a mixed DA agonist (26), stimulated the release of ³H-GABA. The facilitation of GABAergic transmission by ADTN was unchanged when S-Sulpiride, a D2 antagonist (26), was added prior to the ADTN application. On the other hand the effect of ADTN could be blocked by the D1 antagonist, SCH 23390 (20). This first result suggested that the facilitation of GABA release in the striatum by ADTN was mediated by D1 receptors. This interpretation was

Table 1 : Effects of DA agonists and antagonists on the spontaneous release of ³H-GABA in the dorsal striatum of the rat

Drugs	Concentrations (μM)	Number of experiments	³H-GABA release (% of baseline)	
controls (CSF)		16	98 ± 3	
RU 24926	100	4	76 ± 3*	
ADTN	100	6	130 ± 5*	
SKF 38393	10	9	128 ± 11*	
Amphetamine	10	3	123 ± 5*	
S-Sulpiride	10	7	100 ± 10	nS
SCH 23390	10	8	64 ± 3*	
S-Sulpiride + RU 24926	10 100	5	108 ± 9°	
S-Sulpiride + ADTN	10 100	6	120 ± 10*	nS
SCH 23390 + ADTN	10 100	9	96 ± 5°	
S-Sulpiride + Amphetamine	10 100	5	127 ± 13*	nS

The amount of ³H-GABA released during the 30 min drug application was expressed as the percentage of the spontaneous resting ³H-GABA release measured during the 30 min baseline preceding drug application. Values correspond to the mean ± SEM of the change produced by the drug addition. Drug-treated groups were compared to controls using the Mann-Whitney U-test * $p < 0.05$; ns : not significant. The blockade of an agonist effect by an antagonist (added 40 min prior to the agonist application) was established by comparison of the effect produced by the agonist alone using the Mann-Whitney U-test o $p < 0.05$.

substantiated further by the fact that a relatively specific D1 agonist such as SKF 38293 (38) also stimulated the release of ^{3}H-GABA.

Furthermore, when the release of DA was increased by applying Amphetamine, GABAergic transmission was also facilitated. This effect was resistant to S-Sulpiride, suggesting that DA released by Amphetamine may interact primarily with D1 receptors to produce this facilitatory effect.

Interestingly, the D1 antagonist (SCH 23390) by itself produced a marked reduction in ^{3}H-GABA release, whereas the D2 antagonist (S-Sulpiride) was without any effect on the spontaneous release of ^{3}H-GABA. Contrary to the effect produced by amphetamine or by a specific D1 agonist such as SKF 38393, the application of a selective D2 agonist (RU 24926) (12) produced a significant reduction in ^{3}H-GABA release, an effect antagonized by S-Sulpiride.

Although there is no direct evidence for the existence of synaptic contacts between dopaminergic fibres and GABA neurones, some morphological data are in favor of such connections. Tyrosine hydroxylase positive terminals have been found in synaptic contacts with dendritic shafts and dendritic spines of striatal efferent neurones (16), a large proportion of which are GABAergic. The dual effect of DA agonists on ^{3}H-GABA release in the dorsal part of the striatum could reflect a direct interaction of these agonists on GABA neurones and may be attributable to their opposing action on DA-sensitive adenylate cyclase.

Alternatively, the opposing effects of D1 and D2 agonists might result from their interaction on DA receptor subtypes localized selectively on different neuronal populations. In fact, D2 agonists have been shown to reduce the release of acetylcholine and of glutamate, two neurotransmitters which activate striatal neurones. Consequently, the reduction in GABA release produced by a D2 agonist could be due to a dysfacilitation process in the striatum. In the dorsal part of the striatum, however, an indirect effect mediated by cholinergic neurones seems unlikely, since the action of the D2 agonist was not modified by co-application of acetylcholine (data not shown). Furthermore, in the dorsal part of the striatum, the release of ^{3}H-GABA itself was not affected by acetylcholine, suggesting that GABA release in this region is not controlled by cholinergic neurones. On the other hand, an indirect action mediated by cortico-striatal fibres cannot be excluded, since D2 agonists have been shown to reduce the release of glutamate (28), the presumed neurotransmitter of these neurones.

D1 agonists and antagonists, on the other hand, may act directly on GABA neurones. Kainic acid lesions performed in the striatum have indicated that D1 receptors indeed are localized on striatal neurones (10). Since GABA is contained in a large proportion of striatal neurones it can be hypothesized that D1 receptors are, in part, present on this neuronal population. Interestingly, in our experimental conditions, the endogenous release of DA seems to produce a tonic facilitation of ³H-GABA release, an effect unmasked when the D1 antagonist was applied. This facilitation needs not necessarily involve changes in the firing rate of GABA neurones, but instead might result from a presynaptic action of DA on GABA nerve terminals. Based on the fact that striatal lesions reduce DA-sensitive adenylate cyclase in the substantia nigra (31) and that, in this structure, the release of GABA is increased by DA acting on D1 receptors (33), it has been assumed that D1 receptors are localized on the terminals of striato-nigral GABA neurones. By analogy, we suggest that D1 receptors may also be present on recurrent collaterals of striatal efferent GABA neurones. By acting presynaptically on GABAergic nerve terminals, DA released under basal conditions or during some pharmacological treatments such as Amphetamine application would produce a facilitation of the tonic release of GABA, thus contributing to the low neuronal activity observed in the striatum. On the other hand, the D2-receptor mediated inhibition of GABA release might be more phasic and only be involved under specific conditions.

Dorso-Ventral Differences in the Responses Observed in the Striatum

When the effects of various pharmacological treatments on (³H)-GABA release were compared between ventral and dorsal parts of the striatum, several differences emerged. For example, whereas local application of a D1 agonist (SKF 38393) increased the release of ³H-GABA in the dorsal part of the striatum, in the ventral part this D1-agonist reduced ³H-GABA release. Since a relatively homogeneous distribution has been reported for D1-binding sites (35), as well as for DARPP-32 (30), a phosphoprotein restricted to dopaminoceptive neurones, such differences cannot be explained by a heterogeneity in D1 receptor localisation.

Differences between dorsal and ventral regions of the striatum have also been found following other pharmacological treatments. For instance, the D2 agonist RU 24926 was unable to affect ³H-GABA release in the ventral part of the striatum whereas it decreased the release of ³H-GABA in the dorsal part. Conversely, the application of acetylcholine (ACh) in the presence of eserine, increased the release of ³H-GABA in the ventral part of the striatum but not in the dorsal part. The lack of effect of the D2 agonist contrasts with a preferential localization of D2 receptors to the ventrolateral part of the striatum (11). However, it cannot be excluded that in this part of the striatum, the D2 agonist might modify GABA release indirectly in unanesthetized rats. A candidate for such an intermediary might be the cholinergic innervation since ACh very efficiently increases ³H-GABA release in the ventral part of the striatum. As the release of ACh from cholinergic neurones is depressed drastically by anaesthesia (19), so such a kind of regulation could be masked in our experimental conditions. We do not, however, know yet if this is indeed the case. A different anatomical organisation could also explain the differences observed. It should be noted that in vitro the same D2 agonist (RU 24926) has also been shown to increase the veratridine-evoked release of CCK in the dorsal part but not the ventral part of the striatum (26).

Such a distinction between ventral and dorsal striatum is reminiscent of those observed in behavioural experiments following local pharmacological manipulations (1,42). The different biochemical and behavioural effects obtained in the dorsal and the ventral parts of the striatum are likely to reflect a different anatomical organisation in the two regions of the striatum. It would be interesting to know whether the heterogeneity observed in the regulation of GABA release reflects the existence of several subpopulations of GABA neurones involved in different neuronal loops.

MODULATION BY DA OF NIGROTHALAMIC NEURONES IN THE CAT

Neurones located in the substantia nigra pars reticulata (SNR) project to several cerebral regions : the thalamus, the superior colliculus and some other structures (13). Biochemical and electrophysiological studies have indicated that these nigral efferents are GABAergic. Following a kaïnic acid injection in the SNR, glutamic acid decarboxylase activity (the biosynthetic enzyme for GABA) is decreased in the superior colliculus and in the ventro-medial (VM) nucleus of the thalamus (9). These GABAergic nigral efferent neurones exert a tonic inhibitory influence on neurones in their projection areas (8). Blockade of the discharge of the SNR cells by applying GABA or a

GABA agonist in the SNR disinhibited neuronal activity in the VM nucleus and in the intermediate layer of the superior colliculus.

We have examined, the nigral efferent projections of the SNR in the cat by autoradiographic analysis of the anterograde transport of labelled proteins following an injection of a mixture of ^{14}C-amino acids into the SNR. The main projections were found, as expected, to be to the intermediate layer of the superior colliculus, to the VM nucleus and also to the intralaminar nuclei of the thalamus. The VM nucleus was labelled densely after injection of ^{14}C-amino acids into the posterior and ventral parts of the SNR, whereas more dorsal injections labelled preferentially the intralaminar nuclei. In this region, a clustered distribution of radioactivity was observed, the radioactive material being transported to two main zones: the nucleus centralis lateralis (CL) and the paralamellar zone of the nucleus medialis dorsalis (MDpl) plus the nucleus paracentralis (PC), separated by the internal medullar lamina, which was apparently devoid of transported radioactivity (Fig 1).

Since dopaminergic dendrites innervate the SNR, we were interested to know whether the DA released from the distal dendrites could change the activity of nigro-thalamic GABAergic neurones. For this purpose, the release of ³H-GABA was measured in the VM nucleus and the MDpl (zone) of the thalamus and the effects of nigral application of Amphetamine (releasing DA) examined. These experiments were performed on halothane anaesthetized cats implanted with two push-pull cannulae: one in the SNR and a second one in the thalamic nucleus of interest (Fig 1).

A 30 min application of Amphetamine (10^{-6}M) in the SNR produced a 3- to 4-fold increase in the local release of ³H-DA. In the VM nucleus, however, a marked reduction in the release of ³H-GABA was observed during amphetamine application, which persisted after removal of the drug from the superfusion medium (Fig 1). In some experiments, the firing rates of single cells in the nigral area superfused with the push-pull cannula were recorded using a tungsten microelectrode. These cells had the characteristic high firing rate of SNR neurones (8). Amphetamine application (through the push-pull cannula) produced a marked reduction in the spontaneous single unit activity suggesting that DA released from distal dopaminergic dendrites slows the firing rate of SNR nigral cells. Consequently, the reduction in ³H-GABA released from the VM nucleus probably reflects the inhibition of SNR cells.

At first sight, these effects could appear to disagree with other electrophysiological data which

FIG 1: <u>Changes of ³H-GABA release in various thalamic</u>
<u>nuclei evoked by a nigral application of Amphetamine</u>
in the cat

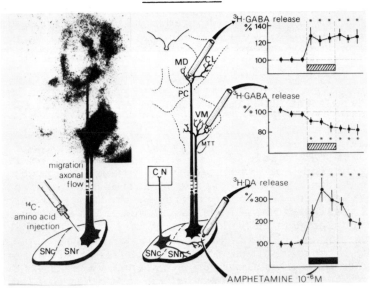

Left part of the figure corresponds to the autoradiogram obtained in the cat from a thalamic coronal
section following a ¹⁴C-amino-acid mixture injection
in the SNR. Middle part illustrates the disposition of
push-pull cannulae implanted in halothane anaesthetized cats; only one push-pull cannula was implanted
either in the VM nucleus or in the MD paralamellar
zone of the thalamus. On the right part are figured
out (from the bottom to the top) the changes in ³H-DA
release induced by an Amphetamine (10^{-6}M) application
in the SNR and the associated changes in ³H-GABA
release evoked in the VM and in the MDpl zone of the
thalamus. Comparison between drug-treated and control
animals (values not represented) were done for each
fraction using the Student's t test *p<0.05.

                    *   *   *

indicate an activation of SNR cells following microiontophoretic application of DA (34,45). However, this
difference could be attributed to the different
methodologies used: in microiontophoretic studies, DA
is applied uniquely in the vicinity of the recorded
cell, whereas in our experiments, Amphetamine applied
through the push-pull cannula has a much larger volume
of diffusion from which DA is released, thus involving
many different neuronal elements. Particularly in
light of the observation that DA acting on DA
receptors on striato-nigral afferents can increase the

release of GABA (33), it is possible that such an effect could inhibit SNR cells, and so mask an eventual activation produce by DA.

In contrast with the inhibitory effects observed in the VM nucleus, the release of ^{3}H-GABA in the MDpl zone was increased by the nigral application of Amphetamine (Fig1).Theses changes do not appear to be correlated with a modification of the firing rate SNR neurones during Amphetamine application. Interestingly, opposite changes in ^{3}H-GABA release have already been observed in both these thalamic nuclei following another nigral pharmacological treatment, application of muscimol (17).

Taken together, all these results call for several comments concerning the neurotransmitter contained in the nigro-MDpl neurones. In the MDpl region, as in other brain areas, the GABA may originate from several different population of neurones and total GABA release is only a global measure of the sum of all these various pools. One of the difficulties raised by this approach is the identification of the neuronal population actually contributing to the changes in GABA release observed. Since SNR cells have been described to be GABA-containing neurones and since the increase in ^{3}H-GABA release detected in the MDpl zone during Amphetamine application is not correlated with SNR cell activity this may suggest that the contribution of a GABAergic nigro-MDpl projection to the total GABA release detected is minor. Under these conditions, the increased release of ^{3}H-GABA could reflect a change in the activity of interneurones or of other GABA afferents such as the afferents originating from the nucleus reticularis of the thalamus (18,41). Alternatively, our results are also consistent with the existence of a non GABAergic nigral projection to the MDpl zone, besides the well characterized nigro-VM GABA pathway.

In conclusion, in the dorsal striatum, DA agonists acting on D1 receptors primarily increased the release of GABA. This effect can also be exerted by spontaneously released DA and in the presence of Amphetamine. It has been suggested that this could be a presynaptic effect on recurrent collaterals of GABA efferent neurones and that it could thus increase the inhibition exerted by these neurones in the striatum. Stimulation of D2 receptors, which reduce the release of GABA, could transiently relieve this control. In the substantia nigra, DA released by Amphetamine from the distal dopaminergic dendrites directly or indirectly inhibited nigral GABA efferent cells projecting to the nucleus ventralis medialis of the thalamus.

ACKNOWLEDGEMENTS
This research has been supported by grants from INSERM, Rhône Poulenc Santé and MIR (83 C 0906).

REFERENCES
1. Arnt,J. 1985 Naunyn-Schmiedeberg's Arch. Pharmacol. 330: 97-104.
2. Bernardi,G. Marciani,M.G. Morocutti,C. Pavone,F. & Stanzione, P. 1978 Neurosci. Lett. 8: 235-240.
3. Björklund,A. & Lindvall,O. 1975 Brain Res. 83: 531-537.
4. Bolam,J.P. Powell,J.F. Wu,S.Y. & Smith,A.D. 1985 J. Comp. Neurol. 237; 1-20.
5. Brown,J.R. & Arbuthnott,G.W. 1983 Neuroscience 10: 349-355.
6. Cheramy,A. Leviel,V. & Glowinski,J. 1981 Nature 289: 537-542.
7. De Belleroche,J. & Gardiner,I.M. 1983 J. Neural. Trans. 58: 153-168.
8. Deniau,J.M. & Chevalier,G. 1984 in Function of the basal ganglia. Ciba Foundation Symposium 107: pp 48-58 Pitman. London.
9. Di Chiara,G. Porceddu,M.L. Morelli,M. Mulas, M.L. & Gessa, G.L. 1979 Brain Res. 176: 273-284.
10. Di Chiara,G. Porceddu,M.L. Spano,P.F. Gessa, G.L. 1977 Brain Res. 130: 374-382.
11. Dubois,A. Scatton,B. 1985 Neurosci.Lett. 57: 7-12
12. Euvrard,C. Premont,J. Oberlander,C. Boissier,J.R. & Bockaert, J. 1979 Naunyn-Schmiedeberg's Arch. Pharmacol. 309: 241-245.
13. Faull,R.L.M. & Mehler,W.R. 1978 Neuroscience 3: 989-1002.
14. Fonnum,F. Gottesfeld,Z. & Grofova,I. 1978 Brain Res. 143: 125-138.
15. Fonnum,D. Storm-Mathiesen,J. & Divac,I. 1981 Neuroscience 6: 863-873.
16. Freund,T.F. Powell,J.F. & Smith,A.D. 1984 Neuroscience 13: 1189-1215.
17. Gauchy,C. Kemel,M.L. Romo,R. Cheramy,A. Glowinski, J. & Besson,M.J. 1983 Neuroscience 10: 781-788.
18. Houser,C.R. Vaughn,J.E. Barber,R.P. & Roberts,E. 1980 Brain Res. 200: 341-354.
19. Jones,B.E. Guyenet,P. Cheramy,A. Gauchy,C. & Glowinski,J. 1973 Brain Res. 64: 355-369.
20. Iorio,L.C. Barnett,A. Leitz,F.H. House,V.P. & Korduba,C.A. 1983 J.Pharm.Exp.Ther. 226: 462-468.
21. Kebabian,J.N. & Calne,D.B. 1979 Nature 277: 93-96.
22. Kim, J.S. Bak,I.J. Hassler,R. & Okada,Y. 1971 Exp. Brain Res. 14: 95-104.
23. Kitai,S.T. Sugimori,M. & Kocsis,J.D. 1976 Exp. Brain Res. 24: 351-363.

24. Koller,K.J. Zaczek,R. & Coyle,J.T. 1984 J. Neurochem. 43: 1136-1142.
25. Lehmann,J. Langer,S.Z. 1983 Neuroscience 10:1105-1120.
26. Meyer,D.K. Holland,A. & Conzelmann,U. 1984 Neurochem. Int. 6: 731-735.
27. Meyer,D.K. & Krauss,J. 1983 Nature 301: 338-340.
28. Mitchell,P.E. & Dogett,N.S. 1980 Life Sci. 26: 2073-2081.
29. Nagy,J.I. Carter,D.A. & Fibiger,H.C. 1978 Brain Res. 158: 15-29.
30. Ouimet,C. Miller,P.E. Hemmings,H.C. Walaas,S.I. & Greengard,P. 1984 J. Neurosci., 4: 111-124.
31. Premont,J. Thierry,A.M. Tassin,J.P. Glowinski, J. Blanc,G. Bockaert,J. 1976 Febs Lett. 68: 99-104.
32. Preston,R.J. Bishop,G.P. & Kitai,S.T. 1980 Brain Res. 183: 253-264.
33. Reubi,J.C. Iversen,L.L. Jessel,T.M. 1977 Nature 268: 652-654.
34. Ruffieux,A. & Schultz,W. 1980 Nature 240-241.
35. Scatton,B. & Dubois,A. 1985 Eur. J. Pharmacol. 11:145-146.
36. Seeman,P. 1981 Pharmacol. Rev. 32: 229-313.
37. Sellstrom,A. & Hamberger,A. 1977 Brain Res. 119: 189-198.
38. Setler,P.E. Sarau,H.M. Zirkig,C.L. & Saunders, M.L. Eur. J. Pharmacol. 50: 419-430.
39. Skirboll,L.R. Grace,A.A. & Bunney,B.S. 1979 Science, 206: 80-82.
40. Sokoloff,P. Martres,M.P. & Schwartz,J.C. 1980 NaunynSchmiedeberg's Arch.Pharmacol.315: 89-102.
41. Steriade,M. Parent,A. & Hada,J. 1984 J. Comp. Neurol. 229: 531-547.
42. Turski,L. Havemann,U. & Kuschinsky,K. 1984 Brain Res. 322: 49-57.
43. Van der Heyden,J.A.M. Venema,K. & Korf,J. 1980 J. Neurochem. 34: 1338-1341.
44. Van der Heyden,J.A.M. Venema,K. & Korf, J. 1980 J. Neurochem. 34: 1648-1653.
45. Waszczak,B. & Walters,J. 1983 Science 220:218-221.
46. Weiss,S. Sebben,M. Garcia-Sainz,J.A. & Bockaert,J. 1985 Mol. Pharmacol. 27: 595-599.
47. Yazulla,S. 1983 Brain Res. 275: 61-74.

Neurotransmitter Interactions in the Basal Ganglia, edited by M. Sandler et al.
Raven Press, New York © 1987.

INTERACTIONS OF NEUROTENSIN WITH DOPAMINE NEURONS
IN THE MAMMALIAN CENTRAL NERVOUS SYSTEM:
FOCUS ON LIMBIC SYSTEM SITES

Charles B. Nemeroff

Departments of Psychiatry and Pharmacology
Duke University Medical Center
Durham, North Carolina 27710
USA

INTRODUCTION

Neurotensin (NT) is a tridecapeptide (pGlu-Leu-Tyr-Glu-Asn-Lys-Pro-Arg-Arg-Pro-Tyr-Ile-Leu-OH) that was discovered in extracts of bovine hypothalamus by Carraway and Leeman (10). Neurotensin fulfils many of the necessary criteria to be considered a central nervous system (CNS) neurotransmitter. The peptide exhibits saturable, specific, high affinity binding to brain membranes (36,39,46,64), is concentrated in the synaptosomal fraction after density gradient centrifugation (65) and is released from brain slices by depolarizing agents via a calcium-dependent process (27). The tridecapeptide produces alterations in neuronal firing rates in several brain areas (54). Enzymes that degrade NT have been identified in brain (see 20 for review).

Little, if any, peripherally administered NT crosses the blood-brain barrier, as is evidenced by the absence of central effects after intravenously administered NT. In contrast, after CNS administration, NT potentiates barbiturate- and ethanol-induced sedation in mice (48), produces hypothermia in several mammals (5), prevents the development of stress-induced gastric ulcers (49), and results in muscle relaxation (55), analgesia (12,56), decreased food consumption (21,41), catalepsy (63), and alterations in locomotor activity (29,30,48). The present review focuses on a review of the neurochemical, neuroanatomical, and behavioral evidence that has led to the hypothesis that NT is an important endogenous modulator of the activity of dopaminergic (DA) systems in the mammalian CNS.

CENTRAL NERVOUS SYSTEM DISTRIBUTION OF NEUROTENSIN AND NEUROTENSIN BINDING SITES

Carraway and Leeman (11) measured NT in the brains of several mammals and the hypothalamus and brainstem each contained 35% of the total NT in brain; the remainder was found in cerebral cortex (17%), thalamus (11%), cerebellum (1%), and pituitary (1%).

Subsequent studies have used both RIA and immunohistochemical methods to elucidate the specific CNS localization of NT. Uhl and Snyder (65) studied the regional distribution of NT in calf and rat brain. Very high concentrations of the tridecapeptide were observed in the medial and anterior hypothalamus, caudate nucleus, globus pallidus, and putamen with lower but measurable quantities in the anterior thalamic nucleus and cerebral cortex.

Combining the microdissection procedure of Palkovits (58) and an RIA, Kobayashi et al. (37) studied the distribution of NT in the rat. Highest concentrations of the tridecapeptide were found in the nucleus accumbens, preoptic area, and mediobasal hypothalamus. In addition to the nucleus accumbens, other limbic structures including the septum and amygdala contained substantial NT-like immunoreactivity.

Uhl and his colleagues have comprehensively described the immunohistochemical distribution of NT in the CNS (see 67 for review). In the mesencephalon, NT staining was seen dorsal to the interpeduncular nucleus and in the substantia nigra, zona compacta. In the diencephalon, the median eminence and preoptic area exhibited dense fluorescence with substantial NT-reactive fibers in the lateral hypothalamus. In the epithalamus, the lateral habenula showed substantial NT positive staining. In the forebrain, the central amygdaloid nucleus, lateral portion of the stria terminalis (and its associated interstitial nucleus), the septum, the nucleus accumbens, and the diagonal band of Broca all displayed dense NT immunoreactivity.

In a subsequent study Uhl et al. (66) utilized colchicine-pretreated rats, which permitted localization in the brainstem of both NT-containing perikarya and nerve terminals. The substantia gelatinosa of the trigeminal nerve nucleus exhibited the highest density of both NT-positive cell bodies and nerve terminals. Cell bodies reactive for NT were also observed in the nucleus of the solitary tract, the parabrachial nuclei, the locus coeruleus, the dorsal raphe nucleus, the periaqueductal gray, and the ventral tegmental area.

Jennes et al. (28) reported that NT-immunoreactivity is widely distributed throughout the brain, especially in forebrain and midbrain limbic structures, but also in the pons, medulla, and spinal cord. The largest collections of NT-containing perikarya were observed in the lateral septum, bed nucleus of the stria terminalis, the diagonal band, paraventricular nucleus, arcuate nucleus, the periventricular nucleus of the thalamus, and the medial and central amygdala. In the lower brainstem, NT-containing cells were observed in the raphe nuclei, locus coeruleus, nucleus of the solitary tract, and in the reticular formation. Neurotensin-containing nerve terminals were seen in all regions that contained NT-positive perikarya and in addition were observed in the cortex, claustrum, caudate-putamen, globus pallidus, nucleus accumbens, thalamic nuclei, and the substantia gelatinosa of the spinal cord. In the cat, Goedert et al. (18) reported that NT-like immunoreactivity in the caudate nucleus, like enkephalin-like immunoreactivity, is found in a patchy distribution. Recently Kohler and Eriksson (38) observed NT-containing perikarya in the lateral and medial septum, the diagonal band of Broca and in the substantia innominata and olfactory tubercle of the rat.

Our group (44,45) has measured NT by RIA in post-mortem brain tissue of humans without neurologic or psychiatric disorders (see Fig. 1). Highest concentrations were present in the hypothalamus, substantia nigra, and limbic areas, whereas lesser amounts were found in cortex and striatum. Cooper et al. (13) have assayed NT by RIA in human brain and have also found high levels in the substantia nigra; other regions that contained the peptide include the globus pallidus and amygdala. Although different RIA methods were used to measure NT in our study and that of Cooper et al. (13), the results were remarkably similar. Ghatei et al. (16) recently measured NT by RIA in the human brain. High concentrations were found in the substantia nigra, periacqueductal gray, septum and hypothalamus.

In the rat, six NT-containing neural circuits have been demonstrated: (1) from cells in the central nucleus of the amygdala to (and through) the bed nucleus of the stria terminalis (67); (2) from cells in the arcuate (and paraventricular) nucleus to the median eminence (24,28); (3) from cells in the ventral tegmental area (VTA) to the nucleus accumbens (34); (4) from cells in the medial nucleus of the amygdala to the ventromedial nucleus of the hypothalamus (25); (5) from cells in the endopiriform nucleus and prepyriform cortex to the anterior olfactory nucleus, the nucleus of the diagonal band and the medio-dorsal thalamic nucleus (26); and (6) from cells in the periaqueductal gray, nucleus of the solitary tract and parabrachial nuclei to the nucleus raphe magnus (4).

The functional interaction between NT and DA neurons could conceivably be exerted at three levels. First, the

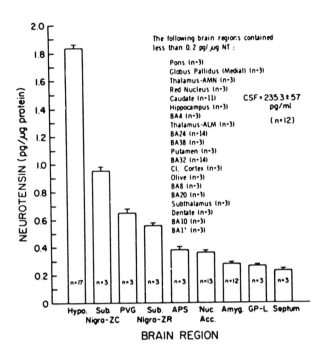

The following brain regions contained less than 0.2 pg/µg NT :

Pons (n=3)
Globus Pallidus (Medial) (n=3)
Thalamus-AMN (n=3)
Red Nucleus (n=3)
Caudate (n=11)
Hippocampus (n=3)
BA4 (n=3)
Thalamus-ALM (n=3)
BA24 (n=14)
BA38 (n=3)
Putamen (n=3)
BA32 (n=14)
Cl. Cortex (n=3)
Olive (n=3)
BA8 (n=3)
BA20 (n=3)
Subthalamus (n=3)
Dentate (n=3)
BA10 (n=3)
BA1' (n=3)

CSF = 235.3 ± 57 pg/ml

(n=12)

FIG. 1. Regional distribution of immunoreactive neurotensin in human brain. Brain areas are presented in order of decreasing concentrations of immunoreactive NT. Cerebrospinal fluid from nonpsychiatric patients contains 235.3 ± 57 pg/ml (n = 12). Values represent means ± SEM and have not been corrected for recoveries. n = Number of subjects. BA = Brodmann's areas of cerebral cortex. (Adapted from 44)

colocalization of NT and DA in the same neuron may reflect co-compartmentation and co-release, and result in modulatory influences on presynaptic mechanisms or postsynaptic consequences. Indeed, combining methods for staining of NT and either DA or its marker, tyrosine hydroxylase has indicated the coexistence of NT and DA in cells in the hypothalamus, the ventral tegmental area (VTA) and the medulla oblongata (22,23). However, the destruction of DA neurons by 6-hydroxydopamine did not result in a concomitant reduction of NT concentration in any brain region examined (Bissette, Kilts, Breese, Knight, and Nemeroff, in preparation). We have also found no reduction in NT concentration in the VTA, nucleus accumbens, substantia nigra or caudate nucleus of patients with Parkinson's disease (with large demonstrable DA depletions) when compared to controls (7). While these apparent discrepancies may reflect methodological differences, more work

Is needed to address the question of the neuronal coexistence of NT and DA before its functional significance is understood. Secondly, NT-containing cells may make synaptic connections with DA neurons at various levels. Thirdly, NT may influence DA neurons by the involvement of interceding neurons. Moreover, any combination of these three mechanisms may be operative in a particular brain region.

Scrutiny of the neuronal mechanisms of the interaction of DA and NT in the CNS is most logically initiated by a study to define those brain regions in which neuroanatomical interaction is plausible. A study of the topographic codistribution of DA and NT would seem to provide neurochemical resolution at the level of individual brain nuclei. The results of such a study conducted in our laboratory support the hypothesis that NT-DA interactions are preferentially expressed in specific DA systems (2). The terminal projections of the mesostriatal, mesocortical and mesolimbic DA systems (40) and the cell bodies of origin (for DA neurons as well as other neurotransmitters) were microdissected (58) and the concentrations of DA and NT determined by on-line trace enrichment high performance liquid chromatography (HPLC) with electrochemical detection (35) and RIA (6), respectively. The correlation between DA and NT was statistically significant (Pearson correlation analyses) in the mesolimbic projections.

These results suggest that the influence of DA neurotransmission on limbic system function may be selectively modulated by NT. Such a hypothesis is consistent with behavioral evidence (see below) in support of a preferential influence of NT on mesolimbic vs. nigrostriatal dopamine neuronal function (50,54). Neurotensin is present in high concentrations in the major cell body regions of monoamine neurotransmitters (e.g. locus coeruleus, raphe nuclei, VTA) as revealed by immunohistochemical and radioimmunoassay experiments, and may modulate the myriad of synapses made by these monoamine projections.

Advances in the field of hormone-receptor and neurotransmitter- receptor interactions have been applied to the study of NT. Uhl et al. (64), utilizing $[^{125}I]$-NT, demonstrated saturable, reversible, high affinity binding to calf and rat brain membranes. Lazarus et al. (39) obtained similar results in rat brain membranes using the same ligand. Subcellular fractionation studies revealed $[^{125}I]$-NT binding to be highest in the synaptosomal fraction. Kitabgi et al. (36), utilizing $[^3H]$-NT as the radioligand, examined NT binding to synaptic membranes from rat brain at $24^\circ C$. Neurotensin binding was found to be specific, saturable, reversible, and of high affinity.

Recently Mazella, Kitabgi, Vincent and their colleagues (46) reported that the ^{125}I-labeled monoiodo derivative of $[Trp^{11}]$-NT binds to rat synaptic membranes in a specific and reversible manner. Two binding sites for this ligand were found to exist; the authors suggested that the low affinity site is the one described in the previous studies, whereas the high affinity site represents a new class of NT receptors.

Using an autoradiographic technique, Young and Kuhar (70,71) observed high densities of NT receptors, often in areas previously shown to contain NT terminals. These regions included the deep layers of the anterior cingulate cortex, interstitial nucleus of the stria terminalis, the substantia nigra (zona compacta), VTA, peraqueductal gray, lateral septum, various amygdaloid nuclei, medial habenular nuclei, nucleus accumbens, and nucleus raphe magnus. Palacios and Kuhar (57) reported that 6-hydroxydopamine-induced destruction of DA neurons in the midbrain is associated with a large loss of NT receptor binding. These data support the hypothesis that DA neurons in the VTA and substantia nigra contain NT receptors (Fig. 2). Further support for this hypothesis has now been provided (61,68). These groups have used different radio-

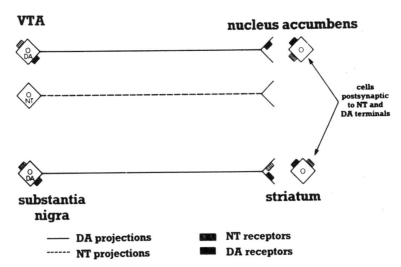

FIG.2. Schematic drawing of selected anatomical relationships between neurotensin (NT) and dopamine (DA). The mesolimbic DA system originates in the ventral tegmental area (A_{10}) with a major projection to the nucleus accumbens. The nigrostriatal DA system originates in the substantia nigra (A_9) and terminates in the striatum. Neurotensin-containing cell bodies and their projections parallel those of the mesolimbic DA system. Neurotensin receptors are present on DA cell bodies in both the A_9 and A_{10} regions and on DA terminals in the striatum. Although it has not been definitely shown, for convenience, we have indicated here that both NT receptors and DA receptors are colocalized in the same cells in the striatum and nucleus accumbens (from 53, with permission).

ligands to demonstrate loss of NT receptors (presumably on DA neurons) in post-mortem substantia nigra of patients with Parkinson's disease.

It is also important to note the report of Quirion et al. (59) who found that, based on neurotoxin lesion studies, NT receptors are contained on the nerve endings of the nigroneostriatal, but not the mesolimbic, DA system.

In summary, the diagram in Fig. 2 illustrates the known anatomical relationship between the mesolimbic and nigroneostriatal DA systems and selected NT-containing perikarya and receptors. The mesolimbic and mesocortical DA systems are comprised of the A_{10} perikarya in the VTA of the midbrain and its terminal projections. The former circuit innervates the nucleus accumbens, olfactory tubercle, amygdala and septum. The latter circuit projects to several cortical areas. The nigroneostriatal DA system is comprised of the A_9 perikarya in the substantia nigra that project to the neostriatum. The VTA contains not only large numbers of DA perikarya but NT-containing cell bodies as well. The VTA also contains substantial numbers of both NT-containing nerve terminals and NT binding sites. As noted above, a high density of NT-binding sites have unequivocally been demonstrated to be present on DA neurons in the VTA and substantia nigra (57). In addition, a NT pathway has been identified which originates in the central nucleus of the amygdala and projects to (and through) the bed nucleus of the stria terminalis (67). The central nucleus of the amygdala receives a substantial DA projection from the VTA (40).

COMPARISON OF THE EFFECTS OF ANTIPSYCHOTIC DRUGS AND NEUROTENSIN

In the introduction I briefly referred to early studies that revealed several similarities between the properties of systemically administered antipsychotic drugs and those of centrally administered NT. Considerable data support the hypothesis that NT possesses a pharmacological profile that resembles that of neuroleptic drugs (35,52,53,54,60). Inhibition of avoidance, but not escape, responding in a discrete-trial, conditioned avoidance paradigm (e.g., shuttle box) has long been utilized as a laboratory screen for antipsychotic activity. Centrally administered NT exerts this effect (42). Intraventricularly administered NT in mice and rats, like neuroleptics, blocks the locomotor hyperactivity induced by indirect DA agonists such as d-amphetamine, methylphenidate and cocaine (50). Recently, we have found that there is selectivity in this action of NT: the peptide does not block scopolamine-induced hyperactivity (62). The locomotor hyperactivity and rearing produced by the three psychomotor stimulants is generally acknowledged to be mediated at mesolimbic DA nerve terminals. Direct injection of NT into the nucleus accumbens, like haloperidol, blocked d-amphetamine-induced locomotion and rearing (14). In contrast, intra-caudate injection of NT did not block d-amphetamine-induced stereotypic behavior; haloperidol was quite potent in this regard. These findings reveal a selective effect of NT on the mesolimbic DA system. Use of another experimental paradigm has yielded similar results. Rats implanted with a VTA electrode will avidly press a lever to obtain rewarding electrical self-stimulation. The rate of responding is reduced by injection of DA receptor antagonists into one of the major terminal areas of the mesolimbic DA system, e.g., the nucleus accumbens, presumably because the rewarding action of DA is blocked at the receptor by antipsychotic drugs. Intra-accumbens injection of NT, like spiperone, reduces the rate of VTA self-stimulation (43). Direct injection of DA into the nucleus accumbens produces locomotion and rearing; NT injection either ICV or directly into this area produces a dose-dependent reduction in both DA-induced behaviors (33). Jolicoeur and his colleagues (29,30) have shown that ICV NT blocks the locomotor hyperactivity induced by the direct DA agonists, n-propylnorapomorphine and ADTN. Such data taken together with neurochemical findings support the view that NT does not act primarily on presynaptic DA nerve terminals in the nucleus accumbens but at post-synaptic sites.

In addition to the data described above concerning the action of NT on the nucleus accumbens, a mesolimbic DA terminal area, we studied the behavioral effects after direct microinjection of NT into the VTA. Bilateral intra-VTA injection of NT produces an increase in locomotion and rearing in the rat (31,32). This effect is consistent with antagonism of the effects of DA released from dendrites in the VTA which normally act on DA autoreceptors. Interestingly, haloperidol has recently been shown to produce similar effects (Maidgement and Marsden, personal communication). Thus although the behavioral effects of intra-VTA and intra-accumbens NT appear discordant, the underlying mechanism of action of NT may be similar at both sites. Scrutiny of this effect of intra-VTA NT revealed that it is dependent on intact DA transmission: either selective destruction of the mesolimbic DA system or haloperidol pretreatment abolished the locomotor stimulation produced by intra-VTA NT. The increase in locomotion and rearing after intra-VTA NT has now been confirmed by Cador et al. (8). The findings of Glimcher et al. (17) concerning the rewarding effects of intra-VTA NT using a conditioned place preference paradigm provide additional evidence for NT-DA interactions in the mesolimbic system.

NEUROCHEMICAL STUDIES

Intracerebroventricular administration of NT, like neuroleptics, has been reported in several studies to increase DA turnover in DA terminal areas as assessed by an increase in DA metabolites, as well as an increase in DOPA accumulation after administration of the DOPA decarboxylase inhibitor, NSD-1015 (50,52,53,54). In these early studies of relatively large brain areas, the effects observed were particularly prominent in mesolimbic terminal fields. It was, therefore, of interest to determine whether enhanced anatomical resolution would reveal a similar specificity of NT effects on biochemically estimated DA neuronal activity in brain regions innervated by different DA systems. Our results of a study in which the effects of IC NT on DA metabolite concentrations were evaluated in micropunched rat brain nuclei support this hypothesis: NT administration produced a significant increase in the concentration of homovanillic acid (HVA) in the nucleus accumbens, olfactory tubercles and anterior caudate nucleus. Of the remaining brain nuclei examined, only the medial prefrontal and cingulate cortex exhibited elevated HVA concentrations in response to NT injection.

After intra-VTA administration the concentrations of DOPAC and HVA, the major DA metabolites, are markedly increased in mesolimbic terminal areas (32); like the behavioral effects observed after intra-VTA injection, this neurochemical effect is abolished by 6-OHDA-induced destruction of this DA circuit.

NT certainly does not appear to simply act as an endogenous DA receptor antagonist, as might be expected. Even in high concentrations, NT does not displace [^{3}H]-spiperone binding from striatal or nucleus accumbens membranes _in vitro_ (50). Moreover IC injections of NT do not alter the subsequent _in vitro_ binding of [^{3}H]spiperone to nucleus accumbens or striatal membranes. The tridecapeptide also does not alter basal or DA-stimulated adenylate cyclase activity in the nucleus accumbens or striatum (50). These results indicate that NT does not interact directly with D_1 or D_2 DA receptors. NT (10 nM) has, however, recently[2] been reported to reduce the affinity of [^{3}H]-N-propylnorapomorphine (a DA agonist) binding to membranes from subcortical limbic structures _in vitro_, (1), though in preliminary experiments we have not confirmed these findings.

The antipsychotic effects of neuroleptic drugs, thought to be due to blockade of DA receptors in the CNS (9), is characterized by a gradually developing, non-tolerating therapeutic effect, and unfortunately is frequently accompanied by unwanted side effects including acute dystonic reactions and akisthesia as well as subsequent tardive dyskinesia. This temporal course of drug action has guided attempts to establish a causal relationship between the neurochemical effects of antipsychotic drugs and their antipsychotic properties and side effects. Moreover, our understanding of the physiology of the various DA systems has led to the postulate that the mesolimbic and mesocortical DA systems mediate, respectively, the antipsychotic effects, and the nigrostriatal DA system the extrapyramidal side effects, of antipsychotics (3,47).

A potentially clinically significant role of NT in the actions of antipsychotic drugs was initiated by the finding of Govoni et al. (19) that the prolonged administration of clinically efficacious antipsychotic drugs produced a significant increase in the concentrations of the tridecapeptide in DA-rich regions of the rat brain. We have found that the effects of different antipsychotic drugs on the concentrations of NT in micropunched brain nuclei exhibit drug subclass and dose regimen-specific effects consistent with their clinical properties (Table 1). Both haloperidol and

TABLE 1. Effects of chronic haloperidol or clozapine administration on the neurotensin concentrations in the caudate nucleus and nucleus accumbens

TREATMENT (14 days)[a]	Neurotensin Concentrations (pg/mg protein)[b]	
	Anterior Caudate	Nucleus Accumbens
Saline (vehicle)	53 ± 10 (8)	287 ± 35 (8)
Haloperidol	164 ± 12* (8)	521 ± 33* (8)
Clozapine	48 ± 5 (7)	414 ± 28* (8)

[a]Either saline (1 ml/kg, haloperidol (1 mg/kg), or clozapine (20 mg/kg) were administered daily by the intraperitoneal route for 14 days and rats killed 24 hours following the last treatment.
[b]Values represent the $\bar{X}$ ± SEM of 7 or 8 determinations (number in parentheses).
*Statistically significantly different from vehicle-injected controls at $p < 0.05$.

clozapine increased the NT concentration of the nucleus accumbens, a terminal projection of the mesolimbic DA system, an effect consistent with their shared properties as antipsychotics. However, haloperidol, but not clozapine, increased the concentration of NT in the anterior caudate nucleus, a terminal projection of the nigrostriatal DA system, a result consistent with its differential liability to induce extrapyramidal side effects (15). Recently, we have studied the effects of the potent DA receptor antagonist,

(+)-butaclamol, and its inactive enantiomer, (-)-butaclamol, on brain NT concentrations. Only the active form of the drug produced increases of NT content in the nucleus accumbens and nucleus caudatus. Although the effects of antipsychotics on the functional dynamics of NT-containing elements cannot be deduced from these data, NT may be involved in the DA system-specific expression of the consequence of prolonged DA receptor blockade.

CLINICAL STUDIES

Because the prevailing theory of schizophrenia remains the DA hyperactivity hypothesis, and because the aforementioned studies provided substantial evidence for NT-DA interactions in the CNS, it was of interest to measure NT by RIA in cerebrospinal fluid (CSF) of schizophrenic patients and normal healthy volunteers. With our Swedish colleagues (69) we measured the concentration of immunoreactive NT in CSF in 21 drug-free schizophrenic patients and 12 age- and sex-matched controls. A subgroup of the schizophrenic patients (n=9) had markedly lower CSF NT concentrations when compared to the remainder of the patients. A second study has yielded similar results (Nemeroff et al., unpublished observations). In post-mortem tissue the concentration of NT has been found to be elevated in schizophrenic patients, when compared to controls, in one area of frontal cortex (Brodmann's area 32) but not in two other cortical areas (BA 12 and BA 24), nucleus accumbens, hypothalamus, amygdala or striatum (51). Post-mortem tissue experiments are often confounded by multiple drug treatments, variable lengths of post-mortem delay, relatively small sample sizes and problems of diagnostic reliability. Finally the CSF studies assume that the concentration of NT measured in CSF reflects extracellular fluid concentrations at relevant synaptic sites and no data are available to answer this question.

CONCLUSIONS

At the present time, it is possible, to formulate a hypothesis concerning the nature of NT-DA interactions. While any speculations are tentative, one potential model for NT modulation of dopaminergic activity is described below.

Considerable evidence indicates that the biochemical and behavioral effects of NT are primarily determined by the neuroanatomical relationship between NT- and DA-containing pathways. If one assumes, heuristically, that wherever NT is injected it will produce effects opposite to those of DA, then the behavioral and neurochemical effects of intracerebral NT can be understood. In the regions that contain DA nerve terminals, DA activity is inhibited by an action of NT at or distal to the DA receptor. In regions in which DA terminals contain NT receptors (e.g. striatum) an additional effect would occur presynaptically. In the VTA, the DA somatodendritic autoreceptors may be blocked by NT resulting in activation of the mesolimbic DA system. In this model (Fig. 2) behavioral effects of opposite sign could be produced by a unitary biochemical mechanism.

Although many questions remain unanswered, considerable progress has been made in understanding the interactions between NT and DA. Both the preclinical and clinical studies strongly support the hypothesis that these two chemical messengers interact with resultant effects on brain neurochemistry and behavior. The possibility that drugs which act on NT receptors might be useful in the treatment of schizophrenia must be explored.

ACKNOWLEDGMENTS

This research has been supported by the National Institute of Mental Health (MH-39415). The author is the recipient of a Nanaline H. Duke Scholarship from Duke University Medical Center. I am grateful to Mary Lassiter and Molly McMullen for preparation of this report.

REFERENCES

1. Agnati, L.F., Fuxe, K., Benfenati, F., and Battistini, N. (1983): Acta Physiol. Scand. 119:459-461.
2. Anderson, C.M., Bissette, G., Nemeroff, C.B., and Kilts, C.D. (1984): Soc. Neurosci. Abs. 10:437.
3. Baldessarini, R.J., and Tarsy, D. (1980): Adv. Biochem. Psychopharmacol. 24:451-455.
4. Beitz, A.J. (1982): J. Neuroscience 2:829-842.
5. Bissette, G., Nemeroff, C.B., Loosen, P.T., Prange, A.J., Jr., and Lipton, M.A. (1976): Nature 267:607-609.
6. Bissette, G., Richardson, C., Kizer, J.S., and Nemeroff, C.B. (1984): J. Neurochem. 43:283-287.
7. Bissette, G., Nemeroff, C.B., Decker, M.W., Kizer, J.S., Agid, Y., and Javoy-Agid, F. (1985): Ann. Neurol. 17:324-328.
8. Cador, M., Kelley, A.E., Le Moal, M., and Stinus, L. (1985): Psychopharmacol. 85:187-196.

9. Carlsson, A. (1978): In: Psychopharmacology: A Generation of Progress, edited by M. A. Lipton, A. DiMascio, and K. F. Killam, pp. 1057-1070. Raven Press, New York.

10. Carraway, R. and Leeman, S.E. (1973): J. Biol. Chem. 248:6854-6861.

11. Carraway, R., and Leeman, S.E. (1976): J. Biol. Chem. 251:7035-7044.

12. Clineschmidt, B.V., and McGuffin, J.C. (1977): Eur. J. Pharmacol. 49:395-396.

13. Cooper, P.E., Fernstrom, M.H., Rorstad, O.P., Leeman, S.E., and Martin, J.B. (1981): Brain Res. 218:219-232.

14. Ervin, G.M., Birkemo, L.S., Nemeroff, C.B., and Prange, A.J. (1981): Nature 291:73-76.

15. Gerlach, J., Thorse, K., and Fog, R. (1975): Psychopharmacol. 40:341-350.

16. Ghatei, M.A., Bloom, S.R., Langerin, H., McGregor, G.P., Lee, Y.C., Adrian, T.E., O'Shaughessy, D.J., Blank, M.A., and Uttenthal, L.O. (1984): Brain Res. 293:101-109.

17. Glimcher, P.W., Margolin, D.H., Giovino, A.A., and Hoebel, B.G. (1984): Brain Res. 291:119-124.

18. Goedert, M., Mantyh, P.W., Hunt, S.P., and Emson, P.C. (1983): Brain Res. 274:176-179.

19. Govoni, S., Hong, J.S., Yang, H-Y.T., and Costa, E. (1980): J. Pharmacol. Exp. Ther. 215:413-417.

20. Griffiths, E.C., McDermott, J.R., and Smith, A.I. (1984): Comp. Biochem. Physiol. 77C:363-366.

21. Hoebel, B.G. (1984): In: Eating and its Disorders, edited by A.J. Stunkard and E. Stellar, pp. 15-38. Raven Press, New York.

22. Hokfelt, T., Everitt, B.J., Theodorsson-Norheim, E., and Goldstein, M. (1984): J. Comp. Neurol. 222:543-559.

23. Ibata, Y., Okamura, F.H., Kawakami, T., Tanaka, M., Obata, H.L., Tsuto, O.T., Terubayashi, H., Yanaihara, C., and Yanaihara, N. (1983): Brain Res. 269:177-179.

24. Ibata, Y., Kawakami, F., Fukui, K., Obata-Tsuto, H.L., Tanaka, M., Kubo, T., Okamura, H., Morimoto, N., Yanaihara, C., and Yanaihara, N. (1984): Brain Res. 302:221-230.

25. Inagaki, S., Yamano, M., Shiosaka, S., Takagi, H., and Tohyama, M. (1983a): Brain Res. 273:229-235.

26. Inagaki, S., Shinoda, K., Kubota, Y., Shiosaka, S., Marsuzaki, T., and Tohyama, M. (1983b): Neurosci. 8:487-493.

27. Iversen, L.L., Iversen, S.D., Bloom, F., Douglas, C., Brown, M., and Vale, W. (1978): Nature 273:161.

28. Jennes, L., Stumpf, W.E., and Kalivas, P.W. (1982): J. Comp. Neurol. 210:211-224.

29. Jolicoeur, F.B., Barbeau, A., Quirion, R., Rioux, F. and St. Pierre, S. (1982): In: Neurotensin, a Brain and Gastrointestinal Peptide, edited by C. B. Nemeroff and

A.J. Prange, Jr., pp. 440–441. New York Academy of Sciences, New York.

30. Jolicoeur, F.B., De Michele, G., and Barbeau, A. (1983): Neurosci. Biobehav. Rev. 7:385–390.

31. Kalivas, P.W., Nemeroff, C.B., and Prange, A.J. (1981): Brain Res. 229:525–529.

32. Kalivas, P.W., Burgess, S.K., Nemeroff, C.B. and Prange, A.J., Jr. (1983): Neurosci. 8:495–505.

33. Kalivas, P.W., Nemeroff, C.B., and Prange, A.J., Jr. (1984): Neurosci. 11:919–930.

34. Kalivas, P.W., and Miller, J.S. (1984): Brain Res. 300:157–160.

35. Kilts, C.D., Bissette, G., Cain, S.T., Skoog, K.M., and Nemeroff, C.B. (1986): In: Dopamine '84, edited by P.J. Roberts. Macmillan Press, London (In press).

36. Kitabgi, P., Carraway, R., Van Rietschoten, J., Granier, C., Morgat, J.L., Mendez, A., Leeman, S., and Freychet, P. (1977): Proc. Natl. Acad. Sci. USA 74:1846–1850.

37. Kobayashi, R.M., Brown, M., and Vale, W. (1977): Brain Res. 126:584–588.

38. Kohler, C., and Eriksson, L.G. (1984): Anat. Embryol. 170:1–10.

39. Lazarus, L.H., Brown, M.R., and Perrin, H.H. (1977): Neuropharmacol. 36:625–629.

40. Lindvall, O., and Bjorklund, A. (1983): In: Chemical Neuroanatomy, edited by P.C. Emson, pp. 229–255. Raven Press, New York.

41. Luttinger, D., King, R.A., Sheppard, D., Strupp, J., Nemeroff, C.B., and Prange, A.J., Jr. (1982): Eur. J. Pharmacol. 81:499–504.

42. Luttinger, D., Nemeroff, C.B., and Prange, A.J., Jr. (1982): Brain Res. 237:183–192.

43. Luttinger, D., Nemeroff, C.B., King, R.A., Ervin, G.N., and Prange, A.J., Jr. (1981): In: The Neurobiology of the Nucleus Accumbens, edited by R.B. Chronister and J.F. DeFrance, pp. 322–332. Haer Institute for Electrophysiological Research, Sebasco, Maine.

44. Manberg, P.J., Youngblood, W.W., Nemeroff, C.B., Rossor, M., Iversen, L.L., Prange, A.J., Jr., and Kizer, J.S. (1982): J. Neurochem. 38:1777–1780.

45. Manberg, P.J., Nemeroff, C.B., Iversen, L.L., Rosser, M.N., Kizer, J.S., and Prange, A.J., Jr. (1982): Ann. N.Y. Acad. Sci. 400:354–367.

46. Mazella, J., Poustis, C., Labbe, C., Checler, F., Kitabgi, P., Granier, C., van Rietschoten, J., and Vincent, J.P. (1983): J. Biol. Chem. 258:3476–3481.

47. Meltzer, H.Y., and Stahl, S.M. (1976): Schizophrenia Bull. 2:19–76.

48. Nemeroff, C.B., Bissette, G., Prange, A.J., Jr., Loosen, P.T., and Lipton, M.A. (1977): Brain Res. 128:485–498.

49. Nemeroff, C.B., Hernandez, D.E., Orlando, R.C., and Prange, A.J., Jr. (1982): _Amer. J. Physiol._ 242:342-346.
50. Nemeroff, C.B., Luttinger, D., Hernandez, D. E., Mailman, R.B., Mason, G.A., Davis, S.D., Widerlov, E., Frye, G.D., Kilts, C.D., Beaumont, K., Breese, G.R., and Prange, A.J., Jr. (1983): _J. Pharmacol. Exp. Ther._ 225:337-345.
51. Nemeroff, C.B., Youngblood, W., Manberg, P.J., Prange, A.J., Jr.,, and Kizer, J.S. (1983): _Science_ 221:972-975.
52. Nemeroff, C.B., Kalivas, P.W., and Prange, A.J., Jr. (1984): In: _Catecholamines: Neuropharmacology and Central Nervous System – Theoretical Aspects,_ edited by E. Usdin, A. Carlsson, A. Dahlstrom and J. Engel, pp. 199-206. Alan R. Liss, New York.
53. Nemeroff, C.B., and Cain, S.T. (1984): _Trends in Pharmacological Sciences_ 6:201-205.
54. Okuma, Y., Fukuda, Y., and Osumi, Y. (1983): _Eur. J. Pharmacol._ 93:27-33.
55. Osbahr, A.J., III, Nemeroff, C.B., Manberg, P.J., and Prange, A.J., Jr. (1979): _Eur. J. Pharmacol._ 54:229-302.
56. Osbahr, A.J., III, Nemeroff, C.B., Luttinger, D., Mason, G.A., and Prange, A.J., Jr. (1981): _J. Pharmacol. Exp. Ther._ 217:645-651.
57. Palacios, J.M., and Kuhar, M.J. (1981): _Nature_ 294:587-589.
58. Palkovits, M. (1973): _Brain Res._ 59:449-450.
59. Quirion, R., Everist, H.D., and Pert, A. (1982): _Soc. Neurosci. Abs._ 8:582.
60. Quirion, R. (1983): _Peptides_ 4:609-615.
61. Sadoul, J.L., Checler, F., Kitabgi, P., Rostene, W., Javoy-Agid, F., and Vincent, J.P. (1984): _Biochem. Biophys. Res. Comm._ 125:395-404.
62. Skoog, K.M., Cain, S.T., and Nemeroff, C.B. (1986): _Neuropharmacol._ (in press).
63. Snidjers, R., Kramarcy, N.R., Hurd, R.W., Nemeroff, C.B., and Dunn, A.J. (1982): _Neuropharmacol._ 21:465-468.
64. Uhl, G.R., Bennett, J.P., Jr., and Snyder, S.H. (1977): _Brain Res._ 130:299-313.
65. Uhl, G.R., and Snyder, S.H. (1977): _Life Sci._ 19:1827-1832.
66. Uhl, G.R., Goodman, R.R., and Snyder, S.H. (1979): _Brain Res._ 167:77-91.
67. Uhl, G.R., and Snyder, S.H. (1981): In: _Neurosecretion and Brain Peptides,_ edited by J.B. Martin, S. Reichlin and K. L. Bick, pp. 87-106. Raven Press, New York.
68. Uhl, G.R., and Kuhar, M.J. (1984): _Nature_ 309:350-352.
69. Widerlov, E., Lindstrom, L.H., Besev, G., Manberg, P.J., Nemeroff, C.B., Breese, G.R., Kizer, J.S., and Prange, A.J., Jr. (1982): _Amer. J. Psychiatr._ 139:1122-1126.

70. Young, W.S., and Kuhar, M.J.   (1979): Eur. J. Pharmacol.
    59:161-163.
71. Young, W.S., and Kuhar, M.J.   (1981): Brain Res.
    206:273-285.

Neurotransmitter Interactions in the Basal Ganglia, edited by M. Sandler et al.
Raven Press, New York © 1987.

PREFERENTIAL STIMULATION OF DOPAMINE RELEASE IN THE

MESOLIMBIC SYSTEM: A COMMON FEATURE OF DRUGS OF ABUSE

G. Di Chiara, A. Imperato and A. Mulas

Institute of Experimental Pharmacology and Toxicology,
University of Cagliari, Cagliari, Italy

INTRODUCTION

It is now well established that drugs of abuse share the ability to act as positive reinforcers (21,23,
29). Thus, laboratory animals quickly learn to self-ad-
minister drugs which are abused by humans (21,23) or
show a preference for that environment where they have
experienced drugs of abuse (place preference)(14,20).
These studies demonstrate that drugs of abuse are rewarding not only in man but also in animals.

The demonstration that animals show towards drugs of
abuse attitudes similar to humans has stimulated a
great deal of experimental research devoted to clarifing
the biological mechanisms involved in the rewarding
properties of drugs of abuse. The fact that drugs of a-
buse are found among the most diverse and apparently an
tithetic drug classes (central depressants, central sti
mulants, narcotic analgesics etc.etc.), would suggest
that each type of drug of abuse acts by a primary mecha
nism different for each one of them. Although this hypo
thesis might turn out to be correct, it does not exclude the possibility that drugs of abuse might secondarily activate a "final common pathway" mediating their re
warding properties. Among central neurotransmitters and
neuromodulators, brain dopamine (DA) has been the major
candidate as the "final common pathway" of the rewarding properties of drugs of abuse (4,29). This hypothesis however is much debated for two main reasons: firstly, while for a drug like amphetamine the effect in
vivo on DA-transmission after systemic administration
is well documented (7), this is not the case for the
majority of drugs of abuse, like opiates, ethanol, ni-

cotine, barbiturates, etc. The reason for this lack of
knowledge can be found in the difficulties inherent in
the in vivo estimation of DA-transmission; on the other
hand, the role of DA in drug-reward has been inferred
from studies on the influence of lesions or pharmacological manipulation of DA-transmission on the rewarding
properties of drugs of abuse in laboratory animals and
these studies have often failed to provide   positive
evidence for a role of DA in drug-induced reward (10,
15,24). It should be pointed out, however, that the failure of lesions of DA-neurons or pharmacological blockade of DA-transmission to reduce the rewarding properties of a given drug does not exclude that DA contributes to its rewarding properties or is important for certain subjective characteristics of the drug-induced reward which are not evaluated by the experimental procedure used for estimating reward. In order to circumvent
these difficulties which in general apply to the analysis of every multifactorial event, one might integrate
the experimental approach with a correlative one, that
is, the study of the relationship between the behavioural effects of drugs of abuse and their effects on DA-
-transmission as evaluated in a variety of conditions
both on a time and on a dose basis.

An approach of this kind has been pursued by us taking advantage of the availability of a method, such as
brain dialysis, enabling the estimation of DA release
as an index of DA-transmission in freely-moving animals
(7,8). Using this method we have correlated the behaviour of the animal to the effect of various drugs on
the release and metabolism of DA in the n.accumbens,
the major terminal area of the mesolimbic DA-system
and in the dorsal caudate, a site of projection of the
nigro-striatal DA-system (27). Interest in comparing
DA-transmission in these two DA-systems derives from
the evidence that they have different functional roles.
Thus, the mesolimbic DA-system has been specifically implicated in certain behavioural syndromes elicited by
dopaminergic stimulants (9) and in the rewarding properties of amphetamine-like and morphine-like drugs
(18,22,25).

METHODS

Male Sprague-Dawley rats (Charles River, 180-200 g)
were used. Each rat was implanted with two dialysis tu-
bes, one in the n.accumbens and the other in the n.cau-
date according to a technique already described by us
(7,8). After the implantation the rats were given food
and water ad libitum and the next day they were utilized for the experiment; on the day of the experiment
the rats were placed in Perspex cylinders (40 cm diame-

ter x 60 cm height) and 20 min samples of dialysate were taken and injected without any purification into an
high performance liquid chromatographe equipped with
reverse phase columns in order to estimate in a single
run, as previously described (7,8), the output of DA
and of its metabolites, dihydroxyphenylacetic acid
(DOPAC) and homovanillic acid (HVA). When a constant
output of DA and metabolites was obtained, the rats were given the various drugs. The behaviour of the animals was video-taped and then analyzed in order to measure the duration of certain behavioural items typical
of the behavioural syndrome elicited by each drug (e.g.
locomotion, grooming, rearing, confined sniffing, lic-
king and gnawing, frozen postures, lying down with eyes
open or with eyes closed, loss of righting reflex etc.).
In order to quantitate behaviour, the duration of each
behavioural item was expressed as % of each time-inter-
val (20 min) spent by the animal in performing each
item. Behavioural items could than be grouped into beha
vioural syndromes and the "intensity" of the syndrome
could be expressed as the cumulative % of time spent by
the animal in performing the items composing the behavioural syndrome.

RESULTS

Amphetamine and cocaine

Doses of 1 mg/kg s.c. of amphetamine sulfate and of
5.0 mg/kg s.c. of cocaine are known to elicit a "robust"
place-preference effect in rats (10,14,25). The effect
of these doses of amphetamine and cocaine on the output
of DA, DOPAC and HVA in the accumbens and in the caudate and on spontaneous behaviour is shown in Figs.1 and
2 respectively. Both amphetamine and cocaine stimulated
DA-release preferentially in the n.accumbens. Amphetamine maximally stimulated DA release by 10 times in the
accumbens and by about 5.5 times in the caudate and cocaine maximally stimulated DA-release by 3.3 times in
the accumbens and by 2.3 times in the caudate. Both amphetamine and cocaine induced behavioural stimulation
characterized by hypermotility and rearing; the intensity of the behavioural stimulation was correlated to
the stimulation of DA-release in the accumbens and in
the caudate.

Opiates: μ-agonists versus k-agonists

Morphine, at doses of 1.0 mg/kg induces strong place-preference (10,14) and stimulates the release of DA
preferentially in the n.accumbens. As shown in Fig.3
this dose of morphine stimulated DA release maximally

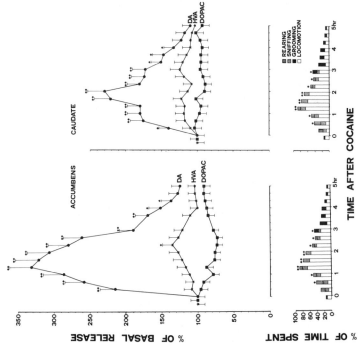

Fig. 1

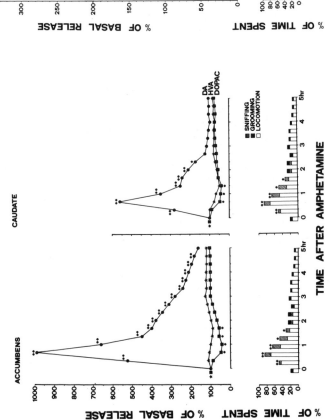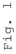

Fig. 2

by 65% in the n.accumbens and failed to affect it in the caudate and elicited behavioural stimulation characterized by fits of locomotion and grooming with rearing. Higher doses of morphine (2.5 mg/kg s.c.) elicited initially motor inhibition with frozen postures and truncal rigidity (opiate-catalepsy) followed by behavioural stimulation and further stimulated DA-release both in the accumbens and in the caudate up to about 100% over basal values. The ability to stimulate DA-release preferentially in the n.accumbens appears a property of other agonists of μ-opiate receptors like methadone and meperidine (see Table 1).

Agonists of k-opiate receptors are devoid of rewarding properties and are actually aversive (13). A selective agonist of k-opiate receptors like U 50,488 (28) reduced by the same extent DA-release in the accumbens and in the caudate and elicited hypomotility (Fig.3). This property was common to other opiate agonists with preferential activity on k-receptors, like tifluadom and bremazocine (19)(see Table 1). Naloxone antagonized the effects of μ-opiate agonists on DA-release and behaviour at doses at least 10 times lower than those which antagonized the effects of k-opiate agonists (results not shown).

TABLE N. 1

Effect of opiate agonists on dopamine (DA) release.

Opiate agonist	Effect on DA-release	Nucleus accumbens	Nucleus caudatus
		ED_{50} mg/kg	
μ-agonists			
Morphine HCl	Increase	0.72	8.5[*]
L-Methadone	Increase	0.54	6.6[*]
Meperidine	Increase	8.5	75.8[*]
k-agonists			
U 50,488	Decrease	1.8	1.6
Bremazocine	Decrease	0.15	0.17
Tifluadom	Decrease	0.75	0.68

[*]p < 0.05 in respect to the ED_{50} obtained in the accumbens.

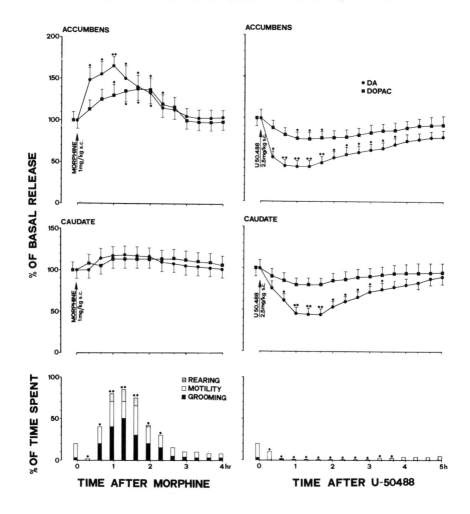

Fig. 3

Ethanol

Ethanol has been shown to induce place-preference in rats, in selected environmental conditions, at doses of 0.5-1.0 g /kg i.p.(17,26). As shown in Fig.4 doses of 0.5 and 2.5 g /kg i.p. of ethanol preferentially stimulate DA-release in the n.accumbens; however, while the dose of 0.5 g /kg elicits a syndrome of behavioural stimulation, that of 2.5 g /kg induces sedation and hypnosis with loss of the righting reflex followed by short lasting motor hyperactivity. The stimulation of DA-release is time-related to the behavioural stimulation after 0.5 g /kg but not after 2.5 g /kg of ethanol. Maximal stimulation of DA-release did not exceed 100% over basal values. Rather large doses of ethanol (5.0 g /kg i.p.) exert biphasic effects on DA-release in the n.accumbens, with an initial inhibition followed by stimulation. There is apparently no relationship between changes in DA release and behaviour except that the maximal reduction of DA release coincides with the period of deepest hypnosis. Administration of low sedative doses of apomorphine, a DA-receptor agonist, abolishes the stimulant effects of low doses of ethanol (0.5 g /kg i.p.) on DA release as well as on behaviour (data not shown). Pretreatment with γ-butyrolactone, an agent which blocks the firing activity of DA-neurons, also prevents the stimulant effect of 0.5 g /kg i.p. of ethanol on DA-release and behaviour (data not shown).

Nicotine

Nicotine is known to induce place-preference at doses of 0.1-0.8 mg/kg s.c.(5). As shown in Fig.5, 0.6 mg/kg s.c. of nicotine stimulated DA-release preferentially in the n.accumbens and elicited a syndrome of behavioural stimulation characterized by marked rearing, locomotion and grooming. Maximal stimulation in the n.accumbens was not higher than 100% over basal values. The effect of nicotine on DA release and behaviour was not influenced by blockade of peripheral nicotine receptors with hexamethonium while it was prevented by an antagonist of central nicotinic receptors such as mecamylamine (data not shown).

Neuroleptics

Agonists of brain DA-receptors (neuroleptics) are not abused by humans. Neuroleptics not only do not elicit reward but block the rewarding properties of typical reinforcers such as amphetamine (25). A classic neuroleptic like haloperidol stimulates DA release both

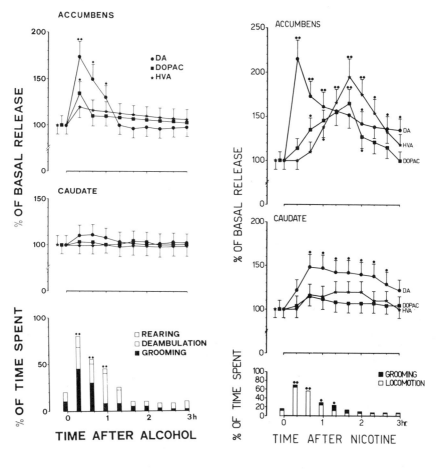

Fig. 4   Fig. 5

in the caudate (8) and in the n.accumbens. However, in
contrast with drugs of abuse, haloperidol similarly stimulates DA release in the two areas and elicits hypomotility and sedation at low and high doses (data not
shown).

DISCUSSION

The present results show that drugs belonging to widely different pharmacological categories but having
in common the characteristic of being rewarding in animals and man share the following properties:
1) Preferential stimulation of DA-release in the mesolimbic DA-system at doses which are rewarding in
   place-preference paradigms.
2) Behavioural stimulation, at low doses.
3) Time-correlation between behavioural stimulation and
   stimulation of DA-release in the n.accumbens, at low
   doses.
The drugs showing these properties range from the ca-
tegory of central stimulants (amphetamine and cocaine)
which act by displacing DA from pre-synaptic sites or
by blocking DA-reuptake to that of narcotic analgesics,
central depressants (ethanol) and cholinergic agonists
(nicotine), which are likely to influence DA release
by stimulating DA-firing (3,6,11,12) through different,
probably indirect mechanisms. A detailed discussion of
the mechanisms whereby these drugs finally stimulate
DA-firing is beyond the scope of the present paper. Here it is sufficient to note that evidence for a role of
DA-firing in the stimulation of DA-release by opiates,
ethanol and nicotine derives from our observation that
agents which impair or block the firing activity of DA-
-neurons like apomorphine and γ-butyrolactone drastically reduce DA-release stimulation by these drugs (see
Results) but not by amphetamine (Imperato and Di Chiara, in preparation). Although at low doses there is a
correlation between stimulation of behaviour and stimulation of DA-release in the accumbens, this is not so
at intermediate doses of drugs like narcotic analgesics and ethanol; at these doses these drugs elicit motor inhibition with rigidity (opiates) or sedation and
hypnosis (ethanol) in spite of the fact that they further stimulate DA-release in the n.accumbens. The reason for this apparent lack of correlation between DA
release and behavioural stimulation might derive from
the fact that opiates and ethanol, by acting at sites
independent from the DA-system and located down stream
to it, interfere with the behavioural expression of increased dopaminergic stimulation. In fact, evidence
from our laboratory (Di Chiara et al., in preparation)
indicates that opiates elicit catalepsy and rigidity

by acting on the periaqueductal grey; ethanol on the other hand, is known to exert widespread central depressant effects.

Drugs without rewarding properties like neuroleptics or with aversive properties like k-opiate receptor agonists are devoid of the properties of drugs of abuse outlined above. Thus, neuroleptics do stimulate DA release in the accumbens but not in a preferential manner as compared to the dorsal caudate. Moreover neuroleptics induce sedation and motor inhibition with catalepsy even at low doses as a result of blockade of post--synaptic DA-receptors. Indeed the stimulation of DA--release induced by neuroleptics does not result in a stimulation of DA-transmission and behaviour because that effect is a feedback response to a primary impairment of DA-transmission through DA-receptor blockade (8). k-Opiate receptor agonists on the other hand reduce DA release by a similar extent in the accumbens and in the caudate and induce sedation and hypomotility.

It appears therefore that among centrally active drugs the ability to act as a rewarding stimulus, to activate motor behaviour and to stimulate DA release in the mesolimbic system are in some way linked to one another. It is unlikely that the rewarding properties of drugs of abuse are secondary to their ability to induce behavioural activation since drugs like opiates, ethanol and barbiturates retain their rewarding properties at doses eliciting a depression of motor behaviour (21,23); these doses however are still able to stimulate DA-release, as shown by our results; we therefore suggest that the rewarding and motor stimulating properties often coincide because they are both dependent, at least in part, upon activation of mesolimbic DA-system. Activation of the mesolimbic DA-system might result in or contribute to an interoceptive, pleasurable effect (reward) and also to a motor stimulant effect whose expression is not essential for experiencing the pleasurable effect. This hypothesis appears in line with a large body of evidence obtained with selective brain lesions and local intracerebral injection of drugs suggesting that the mesolimbic DA-system mediates certain motor syndromes characterized by locomotion, rearing and grooming and that it is a locus of action for the rewarding properties of drugs like the psychomotor stimulants and the opiates (1,2,9,16,18,22,25). We are aware however that much debate does exist over the role of DA and of the mesolimbic DA system in the rewarding properties of drugs of abuse like cocaine and opiates (10,15,24) and that, as regards ethanol and nicotine, specific experiments have still to be performed. One should consider however that negative results after experimental manipulation of the DA-system simply exclude that DA is essential for a certain effect but leave open the possibility that activation of the DA-system is at least one of the multiple factors which contribute to that effect. Thus, although not essential for the rewarding properties of drugs of abuse in general, DA might play some role in drug-induced reward. The fact that, at least in the case of amphetamine, release of DA in the mesolimbic system is essential for its rewarding properties is the basis for postulating that also in the case of opiates, ethanol, nicotine and cocaine, which also release DA in the mesolimbic system, DA adds some still unknown quality to their rewarding properties. Appraisal of the specific "quality" of DA-reward might be the task of future research.

REFERENCES

1. Bozarth,M.A.,and Wise,R.A.(1981):Life Sci.,28:551--555.

2. Bozarth,M.A.,and Wise,R.A.(1981):Life Sci.,29:1881--1886.

3. Clarke,P.B.S.,Hommer,D.W.,Pert,A.,and Skirboll,L.R. (1985):Br.J.Pharmac.,85:827-835.

4. Fibiger,H.C.(1978):Ann.Rev.Pharmacol.Toxicol.,18:37--56.

5. Fudala,P.J.,Teoh,K.W.,and Iwamoto,E.T.(1985):Pharmacol.Biochem.Behav.,22:237-241.

6. Gysling,K.,and Wang,R.Y.(1983):Brain Res.,277:119--127.

7. Imperato,A.,and Di Chiara,G.(1984):J.Neurosci.,4: 966-977.

8. Imperato,A.,and Di Chiara,G.(1985):J.Neurosci.,5: 297-306.

9. Kelly,P.H.,Seviour,P.W.,and Iversen,S.D.(1975):Brain Res.,94:507-522.

10.Mackey,W.B.,and Van der Kooy,D.(1985):Pharmacol.Biochem.Behav.,22:101-105.

11.Matthews,R.T.,and German,D.C.(1984):Neurosci.,11:617--625.

12.Mereu,G.P.,Fadda,F.,and Gessa,G.L.(1984):Brain Res., 292:63-69.

13.Mucha,R.F.,and Herz,A.(1985):Psychopharmacol.,86: 274-280.

14.Mucha,R.F.,Van der Kooy,D.,O'Shaughnessy,M.,and Bucenieks,P.(1982):Brain Res.,243:91-105.

15. Pettit,H.O.,Ettenberg,A.,Bloom,F.E.,and Koob,G.F. (1984):Psychopharmacol.,84:167-173.

16. Phillips,A.G.,and Le Paine,F.G.(1980):Pharmacol. Biochem.Behav.,12:965-968.

17. Reid,L.D.,Hunter,G.A.,Beaman,C.M.,and Hubbell,C.L. (1985):Pharmacol.Biochem.Behav.,22:483-487.

18. Roberts,D.C.S.,Corcoran,M.E.,and Fibiger,H.C.(1977): Pharmacol.Biochem.Behav.,6:615-620.

19. Romer,D.,Buscher,H.,Hill,R.C.,Maurer,R.,Petscher, T.J.,Welle,H.B.A.,Bakel,H.C.C.K.,and Akkerman, A.M.(1980):Life Sci.,27:971-978.

20. Rossi,N.A.,and Reid,L.D.(1976):Physiol.Psychol., 4: 269-274.

21. Schuster,C.R.,and Thompson,T.(1969):Ann.Rev.Phar- macol.,9: 483-502.

22. Schwartz,A.S.,and Marchol,P.L.(1974):Nature,248: 257-258.

23. Spealman,R.D.,and Goldberg,S.R.(1978):Ann.Rev. Pharmacol.Toxicol.,18:313-339.

24. Spyraki,C.,Fibiger,H.C.,and Phillips,A.G.(1982): Brain Res.,253:185-193.

25. Spyraki,C.,Fibiger,H.C.,and Phillips,A.G.(1983): Psychopharmacol.,79:278-283.

26. Stewart,R.B.,and Grupp,L.A.(1985):Psychopharmacol., 87: 43-50.

27. Ungerstedt,U.(1971):Acta Physiol.Scand.,82 : 1-48.

28. Von Voigtlander,P.F.,Lahti,R.A.,and Ludens,J.H. (1983):J.Pharmac.Exp.Ther.,87:481-484.

29. Wise,R.A.,and Bozarth,M.A.(1982):Pharmacol.Biochem. Behav.,17:239-243.

Neurotransmitter Interactions in the Basal Ganglia, edited by M. Sandler et al.
Raven Press, New York © 1987.

PHARMACOLOGICAL INVESTIGATION OF NEUROTRANSMITTER MECHANISMS IN THE BASAL GANGLIA USING THE 2–DEOXYGLUCOSE TECHNIQUE: FOCUS ON THE DOPAMINERGIC SYSTEM

J.M. Palacios and K.H. Wiederhold

Preclinical Research
SANDOZ LTD.
CH–4002 Basle, Switzerland

Many different neurotransmitter mechanisms have been identified in the basal ganglia. Special attention has been paid to the role played by the catecholamine, dopamine, by acetylcholine and by the amino acid γ-aminobutyric acid GABA (2). A relatively large number of natural and synthetic agonist and antagonist molecules for the receptors of these neurotransmitters have been isolated or synthesized. Some of these molecules have found considerable clinical utility in the treatment of neurological and psychiatric diseases where the basal ganglia are thought be involved (6). While the basal ganglia are important targets for these drugs their action involves directly or indirectly these and other brain areas.

Techniques such as immunohistochemistry (3) or receptor autoradiography (9) have been extensively applied to the characterization, at the microscopic level, of the chemoarchitecture of these pathways. However, these techniques provide only a static description of the neurotransmitter interplay in these brain areas. The development by Sokoloff and his colleagues (13) of the 2-^{14}C-deoxyglucose (2DG) autoradiographic method offers a more dynamic way by which to analyze the brain pathways involved in the action of these and other psychotropic drugs, at the resolution of the light-microscope.

This technique is based on the direct relationship between the functional activity and energy consumption of any CNS region and the fact that the brain uses glucose as its main energy source (14). Because centrally acting drugs modify neuronal activity one could assume that drug administration will be followed by modification of brain metabolism and that the pattern of modification would indicate the brain regions involved in the action of a given drug. Descriptions of the effects of a number of drugs belonging to different pharmacological classes are present in the literature (7). These results have clearly indicated the feasibility of using the 2DG technique in drug research. However, only a limited number of drugs of each class have been investigated which makes it difficult to establish comparisons. When we started the experiments described below we asked the following questions: 1) Does the administration of different drugs belonging to a given pharmacological class result in a similar pattern of alteration of regional brain glucose uptake (GU)? 2) Is this pattern of alteration (which we call "2DG-fingerprint") related to the pharmacological activity of the drug, for example, to its interaction with specific receptors? and 3) Is the "2DG-fingerprint" specific for a class of drugs or does the administration of different drugs acting on different systems result in the same "fingerprint"?

Initially we selected the dopaminergic system because of the availability of a large number of drugs acting at different levels of the dopaminergic neuron and of a large body of information on behavioral, biochemical and electrophysiological effects of these drugs and because the 2DG technique has been extensively used in the study of several parameters of the dopaminergic system including lesion and drug effects (7). We looked at the effects of more than 50 different dopaminergic drugs. Some of the compounds studied are summarized on Table I. They included the precursor L-DOPA, inhibitors of the biosynthesis of dopamine (DA), depletors of endogenous DA stores, uptake inhibitors, pre- and postsynaptic agonists, both D_1 and D_2, and postsynaptic antagonists, typical and atypical neuroleptics. The dose dependency of the effects was also investigated and in some cases the effects of other pretreatments were also looked at.

METHODOLOGY

Rats (adult, male Wistar, body weight 280 g) were used in all the experiments. Groups of 4 rats were used per dose and time examined. Drugs were administered generally by the intraperitoneal or subcutaneous routes. A dose of 125 µCi/kg of 2-^{14}C-DG was administered intraperitoneally (8). Animals were sacrificed by decapitation 45 min after isotope administration and the brains rapidly removed, frozen, and processed for autoradiography following standard procedures. Autoradiograms were quantified using a computer-assisted image analysis system. Calibrated plastic standards were

TABLE I

EXAMPLE OF THE DOPAMINERGIC COMPOUNDS STUDIED USING THE 2-DEOXYGLUCOSE TECHNIQUE

DIRECT AGONISTS

D_2 : apomorphine, N-propyl-norapo-morphine, 201-678, 5 OH-DPAT, pergolide, LY 141865, LY 171555, lisuride

D_1 : SKF 38393

PARTIAL/PRESYNAPTIC AGONISTS

transdihydrolisuride (TDHL)
CU 32-085

(−) 3 PPP, TL 99, CF 25397

INDIRECT AGONISTS

L-dopa, d-amphetamine, nomifensine, mazindol

DIRECT ANTAGONISTS

D_2 typical : YM 09151-2, spiperone, haloperidol, pimozide, chlorpromazine, butaclamol

D_2 atypical: clozapine, thioridazine, metochlorpramide, molindone, sulpiride

D_1 : SCH 23390, bulbocapnine

INDIRECT ANTAGONISTS

α-MPT, reserpine

used to transform optical densities into tissue ^{14}C–concentrations. Because we did not measure blood glucose curves we
cannot determine rates of local glucose utilization, but
rather 2–DG uptake. In order to correct for intra–individual
variations in brain glucose uptake, regional values were
divided by the mean brain glucose uptake as measured by
determining the mean ^{14}C–concentrations of whole coronal
sections at different levels. Regional values were compared
with those from vehicle–treated animals and expressed as per
cent values of controls. The computer was programmed to
calculate the individual relative values, mean and standard
deviation from each experimental group as well as to perform
statistical comparisons with control values. Results were
printed and a graphic "profile" was generated along with a
list of the structures measured, mean control values,
statistical analysis of the comparison of the two groups and
as bars, corresponding to each region. The length of the
bars is proportional to the per cent change with respect to
control values and the width indicates the statistical
significance of these comparisons (Fig. 1).

RESULTS AND DISCUSSION

Two general pattern of brain GU modification after administration of dopaminergic drugs emerged from our results. One
was produced by the administration of dopamine receptor
blockers (neuroleptics) and is referred to as the "neuroleptic
2–DG fingerprint". This pattern was also observed after other
treatments leading to decreased or blockade of dopaminergic
neurotransmission. The general pattern of GU modification is
represented by the bar diagram shown in Fig. 1.

The main feature of the "neuroleptic 2–DG fingerprint" was a
marked increase in the GU of the nucleus of the lateral
habenula a component of the epithalamus. Other characteristics were decreases in areas of the thalamus, the
subthalamic nucleus and neocortex and increases on GU in
the nucleus accumbens and substantia nigra compacta (Fig.
2). This pattern of modification of GU utilization was seen
after treatment with "typical" and "atypical" neuroleptics. It
was dose-dependent, presenting a maximal effect, which was
lower for some atypical neuroleptics (clozapine, thioridazine
and sulpiride). The rank order of activity of the neuroleptics corresponded to that of drugs acting on D_2–DA receptors
(Seeman, 1981). The peripheral "neuroleptic" domperidone did
not produce this fingerprint indicating the involvement of
central DA-receptors. Furthermore, this pattern differed from
those produced by drugs belonging to other pharmacological

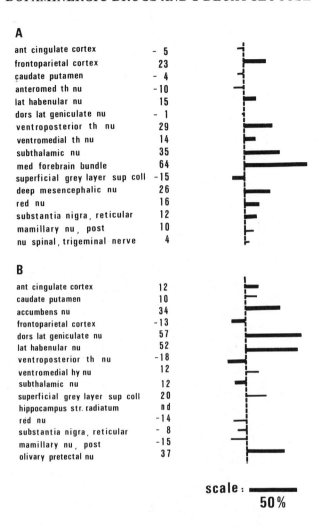

A

ant cingulate cortex	- 5
frontoparietal cortex	23
caudate putamen	- 4
anteromed th nu	-10
lat habenular nu	15
dors lat geniculate nu	- 1
ventroposterior th nu	29
ventromedial th nu	14
subthalamic nu	35
med forebrain bundle	64
superficial grey layer sup coll	-15
deep mesencephalic nu	26
red nu	16
substantia nigra, reticular	12
mamillary nu, post	10
nu spinal, trigeminal nerve	4

B

ant cingulate cortex	12
caudate putamen	10
accumbens nu	34
frontoparietal cortex	-13
dors lat geniculate nu	57
lat habenular nu	52
ventroposterior th nu	-18
ventromedial hy nu	12
subthalamic nu	12
superficial grey layer sup coll	20
hippocampus str. radiatum	n d
red nu	-14
substantia nigra, reticular	- 8
mamillary nu, post	-15
olivary pretectal nu	37

scale: ▬▬▬▬
50%

FIG.1 2-deoxyglucose "fingerprints" from A a DA–D$_2$ receptor agonist (LY 141865) and B an antagonist (spiperone). Changes in GU are given as per cent modification with respect to control (vehicle injected) values as positive indicating an increase over control value or negative indicating a decrease in glucose uptake. Results are represented graphically by the bar diagrams where the length of the bar is proportional to the per cent modification with respect to control, direction indicates increase (right) or decrease (left) and thickness indicates statistical significance P < 0.01 for thicker bars and non-significant for thinner. Results are expressed as the mean of at least 4 animals. S.D. was always smaller than 10 % of the mean value.

groups such as antimuscarinics, serotonin blockers or antihistaminics. Interestingly, other pharmacological manipulations which are known to result in the blockade of dopaminergic neurotransmission also produced a "neuroleptic 2-DG fingerprint". Such was the case after inhibition of DA synthesis with α-methyl-p-tyrosine or DA-depletion with reserpine.

In contrast to the neuroleptics, which tended to decrease the metabolic activity of many brain areas, dopaminergic agonists induced an increase in GU in a large number of brain structures. The main features of the "DA-agonist 2DG fingerprint" are illustrated in Fig. 1. Marked increases in GU were seen in: areas of the neocortex, some thalamic nuclei, the nucleus subthalamicus, a region in the lateral hypothalamus, probably a part of the medial forebrain bundle, and midbrain areas such as the deep mesencephalic nucleus, the red nucleus and the substantia nigra reticulata. The GU uptake in the lateral habenula was, however, decreased by many, but not all, dopaminergic agonists (Fig.2).

As seen previously with the neuroleptics, the "DA-agonist 2DG fingerprint" presented the characteristics of a receptor mediated effect. Thus, the GU modifications were dose-dependent, they showed a maximal effect and the order of activity of the different agents tested correlate with that seen for these agents in other tests reflecting DA-receptor activation. In addition, pretreatment of the animals with an antagonist abolished the "DA-agonist 2DG fingerprint". Treatment with indirectly acting agonists such as the DA uptake blocker, nomifensin, the DA releaser, amphetamine, or the precursor L-DOPA, all of which result in an increased dopaminergic transmission, produced a "DA-agonist 2DG fingerprint". Thus, drugs acting through different mechanisms that result in the same final effect, generate a similar "2DG fingerprint".

The role of DA D_1 and D_2 receptors (4) on the modifications of brain GU induced by the dopaminergic agents was investigated taking advantage of the newly developed compounds LY-141865 (trans-(+)-4,4a,5,6,7,8,8a,9-octahydro-6-propyl-2H-pyrazolo[3,4-g]quinoline diHCl), a specific D_2 agonist; YM-09151-2 (N-[(2RS,3RS)-1-benzyl-2-methyl-3-pyrrol-idinyl]-5-chloro-2-methoxy-4-methylaminobenzamide), a new benzamide neuroleptic which has been described as a specific D_2 antagonist; SKF 38393 (2,3,4,5-tetrahydro-7,8-dihydroxy-1-phenyl-1H-3-benzazepine), a selective, centrally acting D_1 agonist, and the recently described D_1 antagonist SCH 23390 [(R)-(+)-8-chloro-2,3,4,5-tetrahydro-3-methyl-5-phenyl-1H-3-benzazepin-7-ol] (11 and references therein).

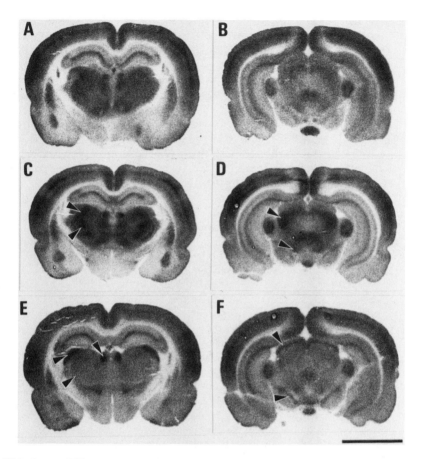

FIG.2 Effects of the administration of the DA–receptor agonist LY 141865 (1 mg/kg) and the antagonist spiperone (0.3 mg/kg) on 2DG uptake in several brain areas. The pictures are photomicrographs from autoradiograms from coronal sections at a midthalamic level (A,C,E) or midbrain (B,D,F) from control animals (A and B) treated with the agonist (C and D) or the antagonist (E and F). Note the increased GU in the ventral thalamus (lower arrow in C), deep mesencephalic nucleus (top arrow in D) and red nucleus (lower arrow in D) induced by the agonist and the increased GU uptake produced by the antagonist in the lateral geniculus (lateral top arrow in E), lateral habenula (lateral top arrow in E), the superior colliculus (top arrow in F) and the substantia nigra compacta (lower arrow in F). Decreased GU was seen after antagonist administration in the ventral thalamus (lower arrow in E). Bar = 5 mm

While the administration of selective DA-D$_2$ compounds produced the modifications in brain GU seen with other active dopaminergic agents administration of the D$_1$ selective agonists SKF 38393 and the antagonist SCH 23390 was not followed by any significant modification of brain glucose metabolism. Thus, it appears that DA-D$_2$ but not D$_1$ receptors are involved in regulation of brain local glucose metabolism.

The activity of compound such as 3-(3-hydroxyphenyl)-N-n-propylpiperidine (3PPP) or the ergot derivative 9,10-didehydro-6-methyl-8β-(2-pyridylthiomethyl)ergoline (CF 25-397) which has been proposed to act at the presynaptic DA-receptor was also investigated (10). Interestingly the administration of these drugs resulted in a "2DG fingerprint", similar to the one observed after neuroleptic treatment, indicating that these compounds could block dopaminergic transmission in the basal ganglia. Other interesting classes of dopaminergic compounds are the "partial" agonists, an example of which is transdihydrolisuride (TDHL). These compounds act in a dualistic mode, behaving like agonists in, for example, decreasing prolactin secretion or inducing contralateral turning behavior in rats bearing unilateral lesions of the striato nigral pathway and as antagonists, in stimulating DA turnover or blocking stereotyped and exploratory behavior (5). The administration of TDHL to rats modified GU in a way similar to the neuroleptics (Palacios and Wiederhold, unpublished results). More interestingly the effects of these and other compounds, was different when studied in a hypersensitive system (1) such as the one resulting from lesions of the striato nigral pathway. In these animals (Fig.3) TDHL and the D$_1$ agonist SKF 38393 produced the 2DG pattern of an agonist in the lesioned side while in the intact side TDHL behaved like an antagonist and the DA-D$_1$ agonist was inactive (Palacios and Wiederhold, in preparation).

Thus, the main conclusion of these studies is that the 2-deoxyglucose technique of Sokoloff et al., 1977 (13) can be used fruitfully in the neuropharmacological analysis of neurotransmitter mechanisms in brain. The technique provides a very high level of anatomical resolution and illustrates the intricate anatomical interconnections involved in brain function. In combination with other techniques with the same anatomical resolution these studies will provide, in the not so distant future, new insights into the mechanism of action of classical and new psychoactive drugs.

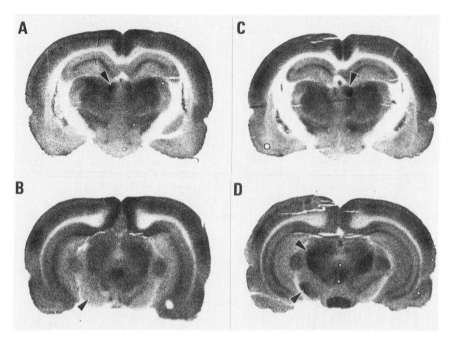

FIG.3   Effects of 6-OH-DA lesions of the substantia nigra on the effects of transdihydrolisuride (TDHL) and the DA-D$_1$ receptor agonist SKF 38393 on brain GU. A and B are autoradiograms from a lesioned animal. The effects of the lesion are an increased GU in the ipsilateral lateral habenula (arrow in A) and decreased GU in the ipsilateral substantia nigra (arrow in B). The treatment with TDHL (C) resulted in a decreased GU in the ipsilateral lateral habenula (an agonistic effect) and increased GU in the contralateral (control) lateral habenula (arrow) as produced by antagonists. SKF 3938 induced increased GU (D) in the ipsilateral substantia nigra (lower arrow) and deep mesencephalic nucleus (top arrow in D) but no effects in the contalateral (control) side. Bar = 5 mm

REFERENCES

1. Carlsson, A. (1983): J. Neural. Transm., 57:309–315.

2. Dray, A. (1980): Prog. Neurobiol., 14:221–335.

3. Hökfelt, T., Johansson, O. and Goldstein, M. (1984): Science, 225:1326–1334.

4. Kebabian, J.W. and Calne, D.B. (1979): Nature, 227:93–96.

5. Kehr, W. (1984): Eur. J. Pharmacol., 97:111–119.

6. Marsden, C.D. (1982): Lancet, 1141–1147.

7. McCulloch, J. (1982): In: Psychopharmacology, edited by L.L. Iversen, S.D. Iversen and S.H. Snyder, pp. 321–410. Plenum Press, New York.

8. Meibach, R.C., Glick, S.D., Ross, D.A., Cox, R. and Maayani, S. (1980): Brain Res., 195:167–176.

9. Palacios, J.M. (1984): J. Receptor Res., 4:633–644.

10. Palacios, J.M. and Wiederhold, K.H. (1984): Neurosci. Lett., 50:223–229.

11. Palacios, J.M. and Wiederhold, K.H. (1985): Brain Res., 327:390–394.

12. Seeman, P. (1981): Pharmacol. Rev., 32:229–313.

13. Sokoloff, L., Reivich, M., Kennedy, C., Des Rosiers, M.H., Patlak, C.S., Pettigrew, K.D., Sakurada, C. and Shinohara, M. (1977): J. Neurochem., 28:13–36.

14. Sokoloff, L. (1980): Neurosci. Res. Prog. Bull., 19:159–210.

Neurotransmitter Interactions in the Basal Ganglia, edited by M. Sandler et al.
Raven Press, New York © 1987.

DOPAMINE AND BEHAVIOR :
FUNCTIONAL AND THEORETICAL CONSIDERATIONS

A. LOUILOT, K. TAGHZOUTI, J.M. DEMINIERE, H. SIMON
and M. LE MOAL.

Laboratoire de Psychobiologie des Comportements
Adaptatifs - INSERM U.259
Domaine de Carreire - Rue Camille Saint-Saëns
33077 Bordeaux Cedex - France

Over the last two decades, mesencephalic dopaminergic neurons have been the subject of extensive
investigations. Anatomical, pharmacological and
behavioral approaches have all been used in attempts
to unravel their function. Dahlström and Fuxe (2)
classified these neurons into dopaminergic A9 and A10
groups on the basis of the localization of their cell
bodies. It was classically considered that the
neurons of the A9 group with their cell bodies in the
substantia nigra give rise to the nigrostriatal
system, while neurons of the A10 group, with their
cell bodies situated in the ventral tegmental area,
give rise to the mesolimbic system (40). The projection areas of these neurons have been precised. Thus
neurons of the A9 group preferentially innervate the
striatum, whereas neurons of the A10 group project to
several forebrain structures : neocortical areas such
as the prefrontal cortex, suprarhinal cortex, limbic
areas such as the amygdala, hippocampus, septum, the
nucleus accumbens and the olfactory tubercle which
make up the ventral striatum (6, 7, 13, 34, 35). The
results of such studies have also suggested that the
distinction between the A9 and A10 groups may be
artificial. It has, for example, been shown that some
parts of striatum are innervated by neurons of the
A10 group (7, 34, 35). The neurons of the A9 and A10
groups may in fact form a mediolateral continuum,
with the dopaminergic mesencephalic neurons forming a
large network which can be subdivided into various
neuronal subunits (7, 30, 34, 35).

Much of the interest in these dopaminergic
neurons derives from clinical studies which have
shown that they may be involved in the etiology of
Parkinson's disease (5), and from suggestions that a

dysfunction of these neurons may underly some psychotic states (36, 37). Furthermore, many studies have shown that dopaminergic neurons are the preferential target of many psychoactive drugs. Dopaminergic transmission is markedly affected by psychostimulant agents such as amphetamine, as well as by antipsychotic drugs (43). The behavioral disturbances that are induced by psychoactive drugs raise questions about the relationship between dopaminergic systems and behavior. Many behavioral investigations have used techniques involving blockade of dopaminergic transmission by local injection of dopaminergic agonists or antagonists (42). Involvement of dopaminergic neurons in the behavioral responses of animals have been more clearly demonstrated using selective lesions of the cell bodies of these neurons. For example, it has been shown (41) that lesions of the substantia nigra lead to a state of aphagia, adipsia and hypokinesia. Lesions of the ventral tegmental area lead to major behavioral deficits. The syndrome is characterized by deficits in basic behaviors required for survival, such as maternal (9), hoarding (20) and social behavior (23) in addition to exploratory and locomotor disturbances (10, 23). All these investigations have indicated the involvement of dopaminergic systems in fundamental mechanisms underpinning behavioral adaptation.

PERMISSIVE ROLE

The extent of the deficits after lesions of dopaminergic nerve cell bodies have led to two opposite views on the role of these neurons : 1) They may be involved in complex information processing during transfer to the projection areas. The deficits would be a reflection of disturbances in both processing and information transfer. 2) Conversely, dopaminergic neurons may not be involved in transfer of specific information, but could facilitate its integration in the projection areas. Deficits would reflect disruption of dopaminergic modulation of processes occurring in these projection areas.

Results from investigations using lesions in the projection areas favor the second hypothesis. Deficits in cognitive functions have been observed after lesions of the dopaminergic terminals in the prefrontal cortex (32). The animals displayed deficits in a delayed alternation task, which is considered to be a sensitive and selective test of frontal cortical function (8, 26). The results obtained in this task showed that lesions of the dopaminergic innervation of the frontal cortex induced behavioral disturbances that were similar to those observed after global lesions of this structure (3). Lesions of dopaminergic terminals of the septum was found to be followed by increased emotional reactivity, shown by enhanced sensitivity to frustative effects. These effects were seen in situations in which the food reward was partially suppressed (38, 39). Similar disturbances have been observed after massive lesions of the septum (14). The two studies mentioned above suggested that the features of the behavioral deficits seen after lesions of the dopaminergic terminals were the same as those observed after lesions of the innervated structure itself. This is also confirmed by studies on lesions of dopaminergic innervation of the nucleus accumbens. This structure has a particular anatomical configuration, it is mainly innervated from limbic structures such as the amygdala and hippocampus (18, 19, 21) and it has projections to the globus pallidus and the substantia nigra (13, 29). These anatomical characteristics suggest that the nucleus accumbens forms an interface between the limbic and striatal sensorimotor systems (27) (Fig.1). Behavioral tests used to investigate the

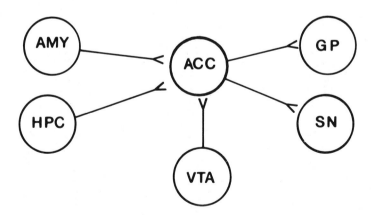

Figure 1 : Schematic diagram of the main afferents and efferents of the nucleus accumbens. AMY: amygdala, ACC: nucleus accumbens, GP: globus pallidus, HPC: hippocampus, SN: substantia nigra, VTA: ventral tegmental area.

effects of lesions of the meso-accumbens demonstrated
disturbances in classical striatal sensorimotor and
limbic functions.

Limbic syndrome

We have used tasks which are widely considered
as tests of limbic system dysfunction (15, 17).
These tests require behavioral flexibility in
switching from one response to another. Two situations were employed using rats with 6-OHDA lesions of
dopaminergic terminals in the nucleus accumbens. The
first used appetitive reinforcement (straight runway)
and the second, aversive reinforcement (passive
avoidance task with foot-shock).

In the first test (Fig.2), food-deprived animals
learned to reach a goal box in a 3 meter long runway
(6 trials per day for 5 days). Reinforcement consisted of two food pellets. On the 6th day the reinforcement was omitted, and latency to reach the goal box

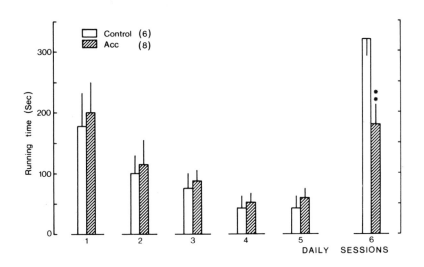

Figure 2 : Straight alley test: acquisition and extinction after
6-OHDA injections in the nucleus accumbens. Latency to reach the
goal box during the 5 days of the acquisition and the day of
extinction (6th day) (mean ± SEM). **p<0.01, Statistical significance with Student's t test.

was recorded every day. Although there was no difference between control and experimental groups in the
acquisition phase $(F(1,14) = 0.79$, NS), on the 6th
day during the extinction phase (6 trials),rats with
lesions continued to run more rapidly (perseveration)
than the controls $(t(13) = 3.15$, $p < 0.01)$

   In the passive avoidance test (Fig.3) during the
three sessions before the foot-shock, the latency to
avoid the platform (i.e. to enter the dark compartment) was identical for the two groups. After the
foot-shock, the latency was increased in both groups.
However, this increase was much less marked in the
experimental group, both 6 and 24 h after the foot-
shock $(U = 22$, $p < 0.05$; and $U = 35$, $p < 0.01$; Mann
Whitney).

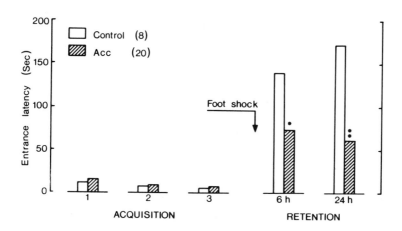

Figure 3 : *Passive avoidance test: acquisition and retention
after 6-OHDA injections in the nucleus accumbens. Median latency
to enter the dark compartment before and after the footshock.
*p<0.05, **p<0.01, Statistical significance with the Mann-
Whitney test.*

Striatal sensorimotor syndrome

   This was evaluated by measuring latency to
initiate a behavioral response in three situations
(open field, two compartment arena and 4-hole box).
In all situations, animals with lesions displayed

increased latency, either to visit the 1st hole in
the 4-hole box, to avoid the central square in the
open field or to visit the 2nd compartment in the two
compartment arena (Fig.4A). However, there was no
difference in spontaneous locomotor activity in a
circular corridor, during the 1st hour of testing or
throughout the 24 h circadian cycle (Fig.4B).

Lesions of dopaminergic innervation of the
nucleus accumbens appear to lead to deficits in the
initiation of the behavioral response which could be
described as a form of perseveration. These disturbances are typically seen after lesions of striatal
and limbic structures. In common with studies of the
deficits after septal and prefrontal lesions, similar
deficits were observed after destruction of the
dopaminergic innervation as after lesions of the
innervated structure itself.

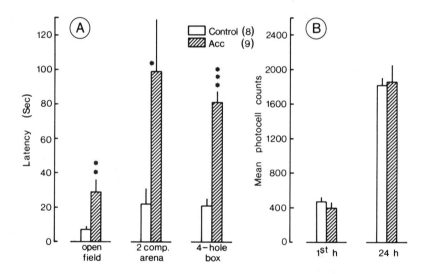

Figure 4 : Effect of 6-OHDA lesions of the dopaminergic terminals in the nucleus accumbens on behavioral initiation and
locomotor response. A) latencies to move from the central square
of the open-field, to visit the second compartment on the
2-compartment arena and to explore the first hole in the 4-hole
test (mean ± SEM). B) Photocell counts in circular corridor
during the 1st h and 24 h cycle of the test (mean ± SEM).
*p<0.05, **p<0.01 Student's t test.

These results strongly support the hypothesis that the dopaminergic neurons have a modulatory influence on the structures they innervate rather than any specific intrinsic function. The partial restoration of normal behavior after treatment with L-DOPA (20) and after mesencephalic cell transplants (4, 28) also supports this view. These results have led to the suggestion (33) that dopaminergic neurons could be classified as regulatory neurons, as opposed to the integrative neurons situated in the projection areas. The integrative neurons can be grouped in different anatomofunctional systems (frontal system, limbic system, striato-limbic system).

The hypothesis proposed by Simon and Le Moal (33) suggested that the various dopaminergic pathways (e.g. mesocortical, meso-accumbens, meso-striatal) do not exert their regulatory action independently but have a coordinated functioning. This would facilitate information transfer from one integrating system to another.

FUNCTIONAL MODALITIES : INTERDEPENDENCE BETWEEN THE DIFFERENT PATHWAYS

We initially investigated functional interdependence between the dopaminergic projection of the nucleus accumbens and the amygdala by pharmacological manipulation of dopaminergic transmission in the amygdala, combined with measurement of dopaminergic activity in the nucleus accumbens (Fig.5). Changes in dopaminergic activity in the nucleus accumbens were studied using in vivo voltammetry, which enables continuous measurement of DOPAC, one of the metabolites of dopamine (11, 12, 24, 25). Dopaminergic transmission in the amygdala was manipulated by local injection of dopaminergic agonists or antagonists. Alteration of dopaminergic transmission in the amygdala was found to have significant effects on activity in the meso-accumbens pathway (Fig.6). The regulatory effect of the dopaminergic meso-amygdala projection on the meso-accumbens projection was found to be inhibitory, since stimulation in the amygdala by the dopamine agonist, amphetamine, reduced dopaminergic activity in the nucleus accumbens, and opposite effects were observed with dopamine antagonists.

The functional interdependence could have behavioral consequences. We investigated this by measurement of the locomotor activity induced by injection of d-amphetamine, after specific 6-OHDA lesions of

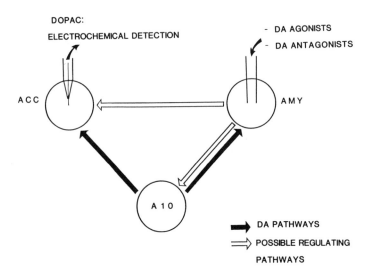

Figure 5 : *Schematic diagram of the procedure used to investigate the functional interdependence between the dopaminergic projection of the amygdala and the nucleus accumbens. Alteration of dopaminergic transmission was achieved by local injection of dopaminergic agonists or antagonists in the amygdala. Dopaminergic activity in the nucleus accumbens was evaluated by the assay   DOPAC levels. DOPAC was electrochemically detected in vivo using carbon fiber microelectrodes (DOPAC : 3,4-dihydroxyphenylacetic acid).*

the dopaminergic pathways in the amygdala. The amphetamine-induced locomotor response is regarded as a good index of dopaminergic activity in the nucleus accumbens (16).

After 6-OHDA lesions of the dopaminergic terminals in the amygdala, we observed increased locomotor activity in a circular corridor (Fig.7). Since local injection of dopaminergic antagonists in the amygdala increased dopaminergic activity in the nucleus accumbens, we supposed that 6-OHDA lesions of the amygdala increased dopamine turnover in the nucleus accumbens. The greater locomotor response to d-amphetamine of experimental animals could be due to increased

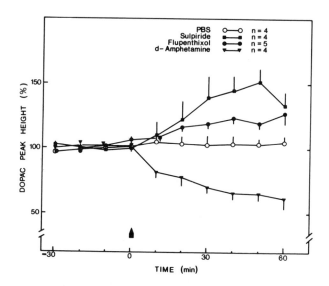

Figure 6 : *DOPAC peak height measured from voltammograms record-*
ed from the nucleus accumbens after local injection of dopami-
nergic agonist (d-amphetamine), antagonists (sulpiride, flupen-
thixol) and solvent (PBS) in the amygdala. Results were express-
ed as the percentage (mean ± SEM) of the respective mean pre-
injection value. The arrow indicates the time of intracerebral
injection (1 μl/3 min). N represents the number of rats per
group. Significant statistical difference observed between
experimental and control groups (ANOVA) : F(1,6) = 23, P<0.01
(d-amphetamine/PBS), F(1,6) = 7.3, P<0.05 (sulpiride/PBS),
F(1,7) = 5.6, P<0.05 (flupenthixol/PBS).

release of dopamine (with respect to controls), since
release of newly synthesized dopamine is known to
occur after amphetamine administration (22).

These results showed the existence of a functional balance between the dopaminergic pathways innervating the amygdala and the nucleus accumbens. It has
been demonstrated that the mesocortical pathway
regulates activity in the meso-accumbens and the
meso-striatal dopaminergic pathways (1, 31). Moreover, current studies in this laboratory shown that
enhanced activity of meso-accumbens pathway led to an
increase in meso-striatal functioning. These conside-
rations suggest that functional interdependence
between these various pathways is a general characteristic of the mesencephalic dopaminergic system.

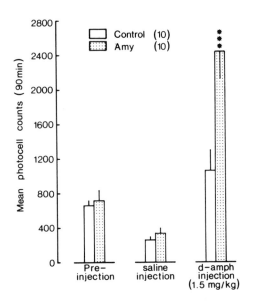

Figure 7 : *Effect of 6-OHDA lesions of dopaminergic innervation of the amygdala on locomotor response to d-amphetamine in circular corridor test. D-amphetamine (1.5 mg/kg) injection was preceded by the habituation period and saline injection response (90 min each) (mean ± SEM). ***P<0.001 Student's t test.*

CONCLUSION

It is suggested that dopaminergic neurons of the mesencephalon facilitate functions in the structures they innervate in a coordinated fashion. It is easy to envisage that such an integrating mechanism could contribute to behavior underlying environmental adaptation. When there is a change in the animal's environment, the following sequences of events could be set in motion : sensory afferents are stimulated, leading to stimulation of the ascending reticular system, which then directly or indirectly stimulates all dopaminergic pathways. This stimulation would facilitate information processing in the various structures innervated by the dopaminergic neurons. One of these integrating structures would be preferentially activated, depending on the exact nature of the task, while regulation of the other dopaminergic pathways would take place via pathways connecting the integrating structures and/or through descending pathways going to the mesencephalon. These processes would thereby regulate the functioning of the integrating structures, especially the nucleus accumbens and striatum which have important connections with the motor system. These mechanisms would increase the probability of the behavioral response appropriate to the particular change in the environment.

Dysfunction in the pathways coordinating the different dopaminergic neurons may therefore lead to similar behavioral deficits as those due to dysfunction in the individual dopaminergic subunits themselves. This possibility may have implications for the etiology of certain psychiatric disorders.

Acknowledgments : The authors wish to thanks Ms. I. Batby and C. Cauchois for secretarial assistance, Ms. M. Kharouby, M. Rivière for technical help. This study was supported by the grant INSERM 133030 and MRT 84-C-1187.

REFERENCES

1. *Carter, C.J. and Pycock,C.J. (1980): Brain Res.,192:163-176*
2. *Dahlström, A., and Fuxe, K. (1964): Acta Physiol. Scand. Suppl.232, 62:1-55.*
3. *Divac, I. (1972): Acta Neurobiol. Exp., 32:461-477.*
4. *Dunnet, S.B., Björklund, A., and Stenevi, U. (1983): T.I.N.S., 61:266-270.*
5. *Ehringer, H., and Hornykiewicz, O. (1960): Klin. Wschr., 38:1236-1239.*
6. *Fallon, J.H., Koziell, D.A., and Moore, R.Y. (1978): J. Comp. Neurol., 180:509-532.*
7. *Fallon,J.H.,and Moore,R.Y.(1978):J.Comp.Neurol.,180:545-580*
8. *Fuster, J.M., editor (1980): The prefrontal cortex. Raven Press, New York.*
9. *Gaffori,O.,and Le Moal,M. (1979): Physiol.Behav.,23:317-323*
10. *Gaffori, O., Le Moal, M., and Stinus, L. (1980): Behav. Brain Res., 1:313-329.*
11. *Gonon, F., Buda, M., Cespuglio, R., Jouvet, M., and Pujol, J.F. (1980): Nature, 136:902-904.*
12. *Gonon, F., Buda, M., Cespuglio, ., Jouvet, M., and Pujol, J.F. (1981): Brain Res., 223:69-80.*
13. *Heimer, L., Switzer, R.D., and Van Hoesen, G.W. (1982): T.I.N.S., 45:83-87.*
14. *Henke, P.G. (1977): J.Comp.Physiol.Psychol., 91:1032-1038*
15. *Isaacson, R.L., editor (1982): The Limbic System, 2nd Ed., Plenum Press, New York.*
16. *Iversen, S.D., and Koob, G.F. (1977): In: Nonstriatal dopaminergic neurons, edited by E. Costa, and G.L. Gessa, pp.209-215. Raven Press, New York.*
17. *Karli, P. (1968): J. Physiol. (Paris), 60:3-148.*

18. Kelley, A.E., and Domesick, V.B. (1982): Neuroscience, 7:2321-2335.
19. Kelley, A.E., Domesick, V.B., and Nauta, W.J.H. (1982): Neuroscience, 7:615-630.
20. Kelley, A.E.,and Stinus,L.(1985):Behav.Neurosci.,99:531-545
21. Krettek, J.E., and Price, I.L. (1978): J. Comp. Neurol., 178:225-254
22. Langer, S.Z., and Arbilla, S. (1984): T.I.P.S., 9:387-390.
23. Le Moal, M., Stinus, L., Simon, H., Tassin, J.P., Thierry, A.M., Blanc, G., Glowinski, J., and Cardo, B. (1977): In: Nonstriatal dopaminergic neurons, edited by E. Costa, and G.L. Gessa, pp.237-245, Raven Press, New York.
24. Louilot, A., Buda, M., Gonon, F., Simon, H., Le Moal, M., and Pujol, J.F. (1985): Neuroscience, 14:775-782.
25. Louilot, A., Gonon, F., Buda, M., Simon, H., Le Moal, M, and Pujol, J.F. (1985): Brain Res., 336:253-263.
26. Markowitsch, H.J., and Pritzel, M. (1977): Psychol. Bull., 14:817-837.
27. Mogenson, G.J., Jones, D.J., and Yim, C.Y. (1980): Prog. Neurobiol., 14:69-97.
28. Nadaud D., Herman, J.P., Simon, H., and Le Moal, M. (1984): Brain Res., 304:137-141.
29. Nauta, W.J.H., Smith, G.P., Faull, R.L.M. and Domesick, V.B. (1978): Neuroscience, 3:385-401.
30. Phillipson, O.T. (1979): J. Comp. Neurol., 187:85-98.
31. Pycock, C.J., Kerwin, R.W., and Carter, C.J. (1980): Nature,286:74-77
32. Simon, H. (1981): J. Physiol. (Paris), 77:81-95.
33. Simon, H., and Le Moal, M., (1984): In : Catecholamines: Neuropharmacology and Central Nervous System. Theoretical Aspects, edited by E. Usdin, A. Carlsson, A. Dahlström, and J. Engel, pp.293-307, Alan R. Liss, Inc., New York.
34. Simon, H., Le Moal, M., and Calas, A. (1979): Brain Res., 178:17-40.
35. Simon, H., Le Moal, M., Galey, D., and Cardo, B. (1976): Brain Res., 115:215-231.
36. Snyder, S.H., Banerjee, S.P., Yamamura, H.I., and Greenberg, D. (1974): Science, 184 :1243-1253.
37. Stevens, J.R. (1979): T.I.N.S., 2:102-105.
38. Taghzouti, K., Le Moal, M., and Simon, H. (1985): Behav. Neurosci., 99:1066-1073.
39. Taghzouti, K., Simon, H., Tazi, A., Dantzer, R., and Le Moal, M. (1985): Behav. Brain Res., 15:1-8.
40. Ungerstedt, U. (1971): Acta Physiol.Scand.,Suppl.367.,1-48.
41. Ungerstedt,U. (1971): Acta Physiol.Scand.,Suppl.367.,95-122
42. Ungerstedt, U. (1979): In: The Neurobiology of Dopamine, edited by A.S. Horn, J. Korf and B.H.C. Westerink, pp.577-596, Academic Press, New York.
43. Westerink, B.H.C. (1979): In: The Neurobiology of Dopamine, edited by A.S. Horn, J. Korf, and B.H.C. Westerink, pp.255-291, Academic Press, New York.

Neurotransmitter Interactions in the Basal Ganglia, edited by M. Sandler et al.
Raven Press, New York © 1987.

MOTOR MANIFESTATIONS OF BASAL GANGLIA DISEASES.
PHARMACOLOGICAL STUDIES IN HUMANS

J.A. Obeso, M.R. Luquin, J. Artieda

Movement Disorders Unit, Neurology Dept. Clínica
Universitaria, University of Navarra Medical
School, Pamplona 31080, Spain

INTRODUCTION

Movement disorders may be divided into two main
categories: akinetic-rigid syndromes, where
slowness and poverty of movement, usually
accompanied by muscle stiffness, are the main
characteristics and dyskinesias, where excessive
and/or inappropriate muscle activity interferes
with voluntary motor acts. Not all movement
disorders arise as a consequence of a basal ganglia
lesion and the majority of the diseases which cause
pathological damage to the basal ganglia also
spread elsewhere. The aim of this review is to
discuss the relevance of the major neurotransmitters and their interactions in humans in
light of recent clinical studies. We shall
therefore concentrate on the movement disorders
which are recognized models of basal ganglia
pathology.

MOVEMENT DISORDERS

Definition and anatomical-biochemical basis (Table 1)

Akinetic-rigid syndrome

Parkinson's disease represents the most common and
best-known example of the akinetic-rigid syndromes.
Other causes within this group of disorders, also
called "parkinsonism", include encephalitis
lethargica, drugs (particularly neuroleptics) ce-
rebro-vascular disease, multiple system atrophies
(olivo-ponto-cerebellar atrophy, progressive supra-
nuclear palsy, strio-nigral degeneration, etc) and
hydrocephalus.

TABLE 1. BASAL GANGLIA DISORDERS: MAIN CHARACTERISTICS

TYPE	AETIOLOGY	PATHOLOGICAL BASIS	BIOCHEMICAL BASIS
Parkinson's disease	Unknown	Substantia nigra (pars compacta) atrophy	Dopamine loss
Huntington's chorea	Hereditary Chromosome 4	Striatal (caudate) and cortical atrophy	Reduction of several neurotransmitters. Dopamine increment
Ballismus	Stroke tumors	Subthalamic and/or afferent-efferent pathways	Enhanced DA activity (?)
Torsion Dystonia	Unknown (a)	Strio-pallido-thalamic Pathways (b) Putamen most commonly involved	Unknown

a. Idiopathic forms. b. Based on cases of symptomatic focal or hemidystonia.

The main clinical manifestations of Parkinson's disease are slow initiation and execution of movement, reduction of spontaneous motor activity, loss of automatisms, rigidity and a characteristic shaking of the limbs ("pill-rolling") in about two-thirds of cases. Loss of pigmented neurons in the zona compacta of the substantia nigra, leading to massive depletion of striatal dopamine concentration constitutes the most significant neurochemical abnormality. Striatal dopaminergic receptors are increased in number in parkinsonian patients not receiving levodopa, indicating denervation hypersensitivity . A significant reduction of 3H-spiperone binding has been found following treatment with levodopa (1). In the early stage of the disease the putamen seems to be preferentially affected, with mild or no involvement of the caudate as assessed by positron emission tomography using (18 F) 6-fluoro-1-dopa (2). Dopamine deficiency may become noticeable only when the loss exceeds 80% of normal striatal concentration (3), indicating the existence of pre and post-synaptic functional compensatory mechanisms (4). In this initial state, symptoms and signs may be confined to one half of the body (hemiparkinsonism).These patients probably represent the best human model of dopaminergic deficit (5). Later in the evolution, the disease spreads beyond the basal ganglia and decreased concentrations of other neurotransmitters, such as noradrenaline (NA) serotonin (5-HT) acetylcholine (ACh), substance P and enkephalins may be detected (6). Earlier suggestions of decreased GABA-receptors and GABA activity has been shown to be erroneous; low levels of glutamic acid decarboxylase resulting from ante mortem anoxia (7).

Dyskinesias

Chorea is characterized by a continuous flow of brief movements in unpredictable sequences, some of which appear to be fragments of normal motor acts. Chorea is usually generalized as in Huntington's disease, but may also be restricted to one half of the body (hemichorea) or one limb.

Extensive morphological and biochemical studies have been carried out in Huntington's disease. The main pathological findings consist of marked atrophy of the caudate nuclei and cerebral cortex. Cell loss, particularly of small neurones, is conspicuous in the caudate and to a lesser extent in the putamen, globus pallidus and subthalamic nuclei (8). In the cortex, the burden of the disease falls on layers 3,5 and 6 of the frontal and parietal lobes. In Huntington's chorea the nigro-striatal DA system is intact. A significant increase in the concentration of dopamine has been found in the putamen, caudate, substantia nigra and accumbens. However, homovanillic acid concentrations are not augmented, indicating that dopamine function itself is not exaggerated in this condition. The current explanation is that dopamine concentration and activity are relativity increased as a result of profound neuronal loss in the striatum (5).

A reduction of glutamic acid decarboxylase levels (GAD) of up to 80% and subsequently of gamma-aminobutyric acid (GABA) concentration is seen in the putamen, caudate and globus pallidus in Huntington's chorea. Thus, striatal choline acetyltransferase levels and the density of muscarinic receptors are abnormally low. Reduction of methionine-enkephalin, substance P, angiotensin converting enzyme and cholecystokinin in the globus pallidus, substantia nigra and/or putamen has been reported (9). In contrast TRH, VIP and somatostatin concentrations in the same basal ganglia regions are normal or slightly increased (9). Most of these changes however, are believed to represent no more than the consequence of extensive neuronal loss involving the pathways utilizing these substances.

Hemiballism-hemichorea.
Hemiballism is characterized by wild, irregular, violent, swinging movements of one half of the body; ballism may also affect two arms or two legs (paraballism) or just one limb (monoballism). There is general agreement that ballism is an exaggeration of chorea. Experimentally it is possible to reproduce hemiballism with great

accuracy by subthalamic lesion (10); but in humans, lesion of other basal ganglia nuclei or their connections (putamen, globus pallidus) and thalamus can also cause hemiballism.

Biochemical pathological studies on brains from patients post-mortem with hemiballism-hemichorea have not yet been done.. Injection of GABA antagonists (picrotoxin or bicuculline) into the subthalamic nucleus in the monkey consistently provoked hemiballism (10), but the same substance placed into the medial globus pallidus did not elicit any abnormal movements. These data suggest that hemiballism may arise as a consequence of disinhibition of pallidal neurons following damage to a GABA mediated subthalamic-pallidal pathway. A role for dopamine in the pathophysiology of hemiballism has also been suggested. Thus, dopamine antagonists are very effective in its treatment and high levels of homovanillic acid in CSF have been found in a few patients, suggesting increased dopamine turnover in this dyskinesia (11).

Dystonia is characterised by inappropriate prolonged muscle contractions which forcefully distort the body into abnormal postures. Clinical and electrophysiological observations have shown that dystonic movements and postures are due to prolonged and exaggerated cocontraction of antagonist muscles, accompanied by recruitment ("overflow") of distant muscles primarily not related to a given movement. No pathological or biochemical abnormality has been identified in idiopathic torsion dystonia. The clinical pharmacology of torsion dystonia is complex and bizarre. Thus it does not provide a clear-cut clue of the biochemical pathology of dystonia. Biochemical analysis of blood, urine and cerebrospinal fluid from patients with idiopathic torsion dystonia have failed to detect any significant change in the major metabolic pathways. Focal lesions of the striatum, globus pallidus and thalamus may cause hemi or focal dystonia indistinguishable from that observed in the idiopathic forms (12). It is presumed therefore that idiopathic torsion dystonia is secondary to some biochemical basal ganglia abnormality, whose nature and characteristics remain to be determined.

Tremor is a rhythmic sinusoidal movement of one part of the body. Three main presentations of tremor may be distinguished in clinical practice: 1) Resting tremor at 4-6 Hz, as in Parkinson's disease, 2) Postural tremor with a frequency ranging from 4 to 12 Hz, as in Benign Essential (hereditary) tremor, 3) Kinetic or intention tremor usually with a main frequency of 3-5 Hz, observed in patients with cerebellar and/or brainstem lesion. It is our opinion, however, that no clear-cut separation can be made among these three types of tremor. Thus, many patients with Parkinson's disease also show postural and intention tremor; resting tremor on the other hand may be occasionally present in patients with benign essential tremor. In addition, resting and kinetic tremors are produced experimentally by the same lesions (13) and parkinsonian, postural or intention tremor can be equally improved by a stereotaxic lesion of the thalamic ventral intermediate (Vim) nucleus (14).

The biochemical-pathological basis of tremor is not a simple one. In humans, the severity of tremor correlates well with the degree of dopamine loss in the striatum. However animal models reveal a more complex interaction. Lesions involving the midbrain ventromedial tegmental area in monkeys produce a resting tremor of similar characteristics to that in Parkinson's disease. A lesion restricted to the substantia nigra has no effect however. Lesions confined to the dento-rubro-thalamic pathway may cause ataxia, but no tremor by itself, unless the animals are treated with antidopaminergic drugs (15). Neurochemical analysis from these experiments showed that a lesion of the ventromedial tegmental area, which damages the substantia nigra and its efferent, as well as the rubro-spinal fibres and the brachium conjunctivum partially, induces tremor by provoking a massive fall in both dopamine and 5-HT concentration. Reduction of either neurotransmitter alone does not elicit tremor (16).

The clinical pharmacology of tremor also has complex interactions. Dopamine agonists may ameliorate parkinsonian tremor, but treatment with anticholinergics is often necessary. Postural tremor may respond to B-adrenergic receptor antagonists and 5-HTP therapy may improve cerebellar tremor. Isoniazid may also reduce kinetic tremor in patients with multiple sclerosis. In practice, polytherapy including these and other drugs is required in patients with a combination of different types of tremor.

Tics and myoclonus are rapid muscle jerks which do not represent good models of basal ganglia disorders according to the present evidence.

DOPAMINERGIC DEFICIT

Loss of nigrostriatal dopaminergic neurons accounts for most of the cardinal motor manifestations of Parkinson's disease. Although there is still debate as to whether the physiological action of dopamine input into the striatum is excitatory or inhibitory, the result of removing such influence is mainly expressed as slowness of movement. Akinesia is the most representative feature of striatal dopaminergic deficiency.

Normal voluntary movements involve several mechanisms, some of which are disrupted in Parkinson's disease. Voluntary movement may be divided in three main stages: a) The idea or concept of moving (motor plan), which requires accurate perception of the external environment as well as knowledge of the physical situation of the body part to be moved. b). Selection and adequation of the motor programs forming the motor plan. c). Initiation and orderly and timely concatenated execution of the motor programs. The anatomical-physiological basis of each of these processes is not completely defined yet. In Parkinson's disease no overt perceptive disorder has been shown and the preparation to move is correct (17). On the other hand, the final motor pathway (cortico-spinal tract) in charge of executing the motor commands seems to be entirely

Table 2. Pharmacological characterization of main basal ganglia
disorders

	Parkinson Disease	Chorea	Ballismus	Dystonia
DA Ago.	↑ ↑	↑ ↓	↓ ↓	↑
Ant.	↓ ↓	↑ ↑	↑ ↑	↑ ↑
GABA Ago.	=	=		=
ACh Ago.	↓	=	?	=
Ant.	↑	↓		↑
5 HTP Ago.	↓	=	=	=
Ant.	=	?	?	=
Usual drug treatment	levodopa anticholinergics ergots	neuroleptics tetrabenazine	neuroleptics tetrabenazine	combination of anticholinergics neuroleptics and tetrabenazine

Table 3. Mechanisms involved in dyskinesias induced by levodopa
in Parkinson's disease

	Type	Presentation
Hyperstimulation of DA receptors	Chorea Athetosis Myoclonus	Benefit of dose
Hypostimulation of DA receptors	Myorhythmia Ballismus	Diphasic
	Dystonic postures	"Off"periods

Legend for figures

TOP.   Very disabling, alternating movement of
          the left leg during the beginning of
          action of a levodopa dose.

BOTTOM.   EMG tracing from the same patient showing
          rhythmical alternating activity at 5 Hz in
          the upper limb (first two channels) and at
          3 Hz. (four bottom channels) in the lower
          limb.

Legend for figures
appears at bottom
of facing page.

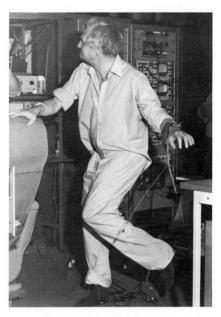

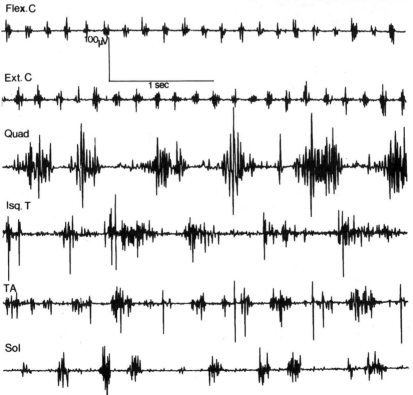

normal. The main abnormalities found in akinetic patients are: 1). Inability to specify the correct amount of muscle contraction required to initiate and execute a movement at a certain speed to a given distance ("energization"). 2). Slowness and fatigue on repetitive action. 3). Inability or difficulty to perform concurrent action. 4). Interruption of action ("freezing") by external stimuli. All of these features are greatly improved or for the most part completely corrected by appropriate treatment with levodopa and/or postsynaptic dopamine agonists (lisuride, pergolide, etc). It is therefore reasonable to conclude that akinesia is mainly a defect in the specification and assembling of motor programs as a result of striatal (putamen in particular) dysfunction, secondary to decreased dopaminergic imput.

DOPAMINERGIC HYPERACTIVITY

Primary overactivity of the DA ascending systems has not been described in any movement disorder. Excessive dopaminergic stimulation exists in Huntington's chorea as a result of loss of striatal cholinergic neurons. Typical chorea is also frequently observed in parkinsonian patients treated with excessive amount of levodopa (Table 3). There is no clear-cut evidence for an abnormality of dopamine in ballism and torsion dystonia. In these two conditions, antidopaminergic drugs, like tetrabenazine (pre-synaptic depletion) or neuroleptics (post-synaptic blockade) probably act by turning "off" the activity of the strio-pallidal complex, so that abnormal movements are ameliorated or disappear because the main basal ganglia output to the pre-frontal-motor cortex is reduced. This often occurs at the expense of creating a parkinsonian syndrome.

Clinical pharmacology: Conclusions

Treatment of movement disorders with serotonin precursors or agonists and GABAergic drugs produces very little modification (Table 2). The massive dopaminergic nigro-striatal pathway serves a pivotal role in normal striatal activity, which in humans is mainly related to movement control (17). The beneficial effects of anticholinergic drugs in the treatment of Parkinson's disease and perhaps in torsion dystonia (Table 2) indicate a dopaminergic-cholinergic balance, which is the predominant relationship among neurotransmitters in the human striatum. However, the influence of the dopaminergic system may not be completely non specific ("on-off").

The study of parkinsonian patients with dyskinesias provoked by treatment with levodopa (Table 3) indicates that partial stimulation of DA receptors may give rise to fragments of normal movements (Figure) or dystonic postures. Even more, in these patients one part of the body may show chorea (hyperactivation) and another may be paralyzed (DA deficit) or suffer myorhythmic-ballistic movements (hypostimulation). It is conceivable therefore, that different types and/or topographical distribution of striatal DA receptors serve to exert a discriminative regulatory action of neuronal activity in the striatum. Surprisingly, the many alternative interactions with other neurotransmitters and neuromodulators at this level do not seem to have any pathophysiological consequence.

References

1. RINNE UF, LONNBERG P, KOSKINEN V (1981). Dopamine receptors in the parkinson brain. J. Neural Trans. 51:97-109.

2. NAHMIAS C, GARNETT ES, FIRNAU G, LANG A (1985): Striatal dopamine distribution in parkinsonian patients during life. J. Neurol. Sci. 69:223-230.

3. HORNYKIEWICZ O (1973): Dopamine in the basal ganglia: Its role and therapeutic implications. Br. Med. Bull. 29:172-178.

4. AGID I, JAVOY F, GLOWINSKI J (1973): Hyperactivity of remaining dopaminergic neurons after partial destruction of the nigro-striatal dopaminergic system in the rat. Nature, 245:150-151.

5. MARSDEN CD (1984): Motor disorders in basal ganglia disease. Human Neurobiol. 2:245-250.

6. HORNYKIEWICZ O (1982): Brain neurotransmmitter changes in Parkinson's disease. In Movement Disorders, edited by CD Marsden and S. Fahn, pp. 41-58. Butterworth, London.

7. AGID Y, PLOSKA A, MONFORT JC, JAVOY-AGID F (1984): Striatal glutamate decarboxylase values, indicative of hospital where patient died. Lancet 1:280, 1984.

8. LANGE H, THORNER G, HOPF A AND SCHRODER KF (1976): Morphometric studies of the neuropathological changes in choreatic disease. J. Neurol. Sci. 28: 405-425.

9. EMSON PC, ARREGUI A, CIEMENT-JONES V, SANBERG BEB and ROSSOR M (1980): Regional distribution of methionine-enkephalin and substante P like immunoreactivily in normal human brain and in Huntington's disease. Brain Res., 199:147-169.

10. CROSSMAN AR, SAMBROOK MA, JACKSON A (1984): Experimental hemichorea/hemiballismus in the monkey. Brain 107:579-596.

11. KOLLER WC, WEINER WJ, NAUSIEDA PA, KLAWANS HL (1979): Pharmacology of ballism. In Clinical Neuropharmacology, Vol. 4, 157-174, Raven Press, New York.

12. MARSDEN CD, OBESO JA, ZARRANZ JJ, LANG AM (1985): The anatomical basis of symptomatic hemidystonia. Brain. vol. 108, Part II, 1985, 463-483

13. LAMARRE Y (1975): Tremorogenic mechanisms in primates. Adv. Neurol. 10:23-34.

14. NARABAYASHI H (1982): Surgical approach to tremor. In Movement Disorders, edited by CD Marsden and S Fahn, pp.292-299. Butterworth, London

15. PECHADRE JC, LAROCHELLE L, POIRIER LJ (1976): Parkinsonian akinesia, rigidity and tremor in the monkey: histopathological and neuropharmacological study. J. Neurol. Sci. 28:147-57.

16. SOURKES TL, POIRIER LJ (1966): Neurochemical basis of tremor and other disorders of movement. Can. Med. Assoc. J. 94:53-60.

17 MARSDEN CD (1982): The mysterious motor function of the basal ganglia. Neurology, 32:514-539.

Neurotransmitter Interactions in the Basal Ganglia, edited by M. Sandler et al.
Raven Press, New York © 1987.

MOLECULAR CHARACTERIZATION OF DOPAMINE RECEPTORS

Pierre M. Laduron

Department of Biochemical Pharmacology,
Janssen Pharmaceutica,
B-2340 Beerse, Belgium

INTRODUCTION

"Classical" neurotransmitters (AcH, DA, NA, 5HT, ...) only possess a low affinity for receptors and are thus inappropriate ligands for the in vitro binding studies. This also explains why the biochemical identification of dopamine receptors has been closely associated with the development of neuroleptic drugs. Haloperidol but mostly spiperone are the ligands that were used to isolate the dopamine receptor. They label the D_2 site (10, 12, 27) which may be called a receptor site because all the physiological, pharmacological and clinical responses to dopamine agonists and antagonists can only be explained by an interaction in the brain on these sites (12). More than 17 biological parameters were found to nicely correlate with the binding on the D_2 receptor sites (12, 13, 20, 27). By contrast, such a correlation has never be found for the other subtypes including even the D_1 site (13) which is the dopamine-sensitive adenylate cyclase (10). More than 10 years after its discovery, this enzyme is still in search of a function; therefore it is still premature to call it a receptor (14). The secretion of parathormone in the bovine parathyroid gland which seems to be mediated through D_1 sites has been repeatedly presented as direct evidence for a physiological role of dopamine-sensitive adenylate cyclase (28). Unfortunately, this effect is purely anecdotal : it is restricted to one species and has not been clearly demonstrated in vivo. Moreover, in human, the parathyroid gland is unresponsive to dopamine and to neuroleptic drugs especially those, like thioxanthene and phenothiazine derivatives which have potent effects on the D_1 site (14). Recently ^{3}H-flupenthixol and ^{3}H-pifluthixol were reported to bind on D_1 sites (9); this was somewhat surprising owing to the lack of specificity of these drugs that bind with high affinity on D_1 sites but also on D_2, α_1 and H_1 sites (9). In fact the correlation between the binding and the inhibition of dopamine-sensitive adenylate cyclase was poor (9) and both are now known to represent different molecular entities (23).

The dopamine receptor has not resisted the rush to multiple "receptor" sites. Five years ago, I wrote about the dopamine receptor "... the postulated existence of the subtypes D_1, D_2, D_3 ... or even D_4, D_5, D_6 ... is probably a short-lived fashion" (12). This prediction seems to come true since even Seeman and Creese who have been in favor of multiple sites and have revisited many times the nomenclature of dopamine receptors no longer believe in the D_3 and D_4 sites as separate entities (18, 27). The fact that they now call D_4 the high affinity sites of D_2 and D_3 the high affinity of D_1 (18, 27) is simply a penultimate step before definitively reaching a more unitary concept.

In this paper, we will discuss some aspects dealing with the solubilization, the photoaffinity labelling and the molecular characterization of dopamine D_2 receptors.

SOLUBILIZATION

The first attempts to obtain dopamine receptors in a molecularly dispersed form were not very encouraging (6); ^{3}H-spiperone binding sites solubilized from rat striatum by means of 1 % digitonin had lost high affinity for all the dopamine antagonists except spiperone. The reasons for such a failure are now known: only spirodecanone sites labelled with ^{3}H-spiperone (a non-specific but displaceable site) were obtained in solution and as they were present in excess they masked the dopamine receptors. The choice of another animal species, the dog, which apparently is devoid of spirodecanone sites, was quite decisive. Indeed the first solubilization of high affinity dopamine receptors was obtained from striatal membranes of dog brain using 1 % digitonin (7). Thereafter, the concomitant use of a more sensitive technique to reveal soluble receptors, the charcoal procedure, and a spirodecanone site blocker (R 5260) also enabled us to obtain dopamine receptors in molecularly dispersed form from rat striatum (8). Since then the solubilization of dopamine receptors has been confirmed by different groups in various species and using different mild detergents (4, 5, 16, 17, 19, 29). The dopamine receptor must be regarded as an intrinsic protein, since high salt concentrations may not be used as the solubilizing agent (15).

Initially, the yield of soluble receptors was not very high; using digitonin it was only 18 % in dog (7) and 20-25 % in human striatum (4). More recently a mixture of cholate and sodium chloride allowed us to get a yield higher than 50 % (cf· Table 1). A value of 85 % was also reported when 1 % lysolecithin was used as detergent (19); unfortunately the characterization of solubilized ^{3}H-spiperone binding sites was not performed with this concentration of lysolecithin but with 0.25 % which gave a much lower yield.

TABLE 1.   Solubilization of brain dopamine receptors in various species using different mild detergents

Detergent	Species	Yield	Reference
Digitonin 1 %	Dog	18 %	(7)
	Rat	–	(8)
	Human	20-25 %	(4)
Lysolecithin 0.1 %	Bovine	10 %	(29)
CHAPS 10 mM	Rat	30 %	(5)
Cholate 0.2 % + NaCl 1 M	Bovine	40 %	(29)
Cholate 0.3 % + NaCl 1.4 M	Rat	46 %	(32)
	Dog	53 %	(32)
	Human	52 %	(32)

PHARMACOLOGICAL CHARACTERIZATION

In order to assess whether ^{3}H-spiperone binding sites sol-ubilized with mild detergents possess all the high affinity characteristics of dopamine receptors, various criteria must be fulfilled (15); among these, drug displacement and the correla-tion with the drug affinity obtained on membrane preparations and with the drug potency obtained in vivo from pharmacological tests are the most important.   Fig. 1 shows the competition of eight compounds belonging to different classes of drugs in ^{3}H-spiperone binding, using a cholate extract from dog striata. Interestingly the non-displaceable binding was very low; it did not exceed 10 % of the total binding and was the same with all the compounds.   Spiperone, benperidol (a butyrophenone without spirodecanone moiety) and (+)butaclamol were found to compete at the nanomolar range.   In contrast, (-)butaclamol and (+)sul-piride, which are both pharmacologically inactive enantiomers, displaced in the micromolar range as did pipamperone, a butyro-phenone endowed with antiserotonergic properties.   Note that the stereospecific binding ratio between (+) and (-)butaclamol was higher than 1,000-fold.

In brain soluble extract, ^{3}H-spiperone was found to bind to at least three different sites; the dopamine D_2 receptor, the serotonin S_2 receptor and the spirodecanone site.   The latter is a displaceable binding site without any physiological relevance.   The ^{3}H-spiperone binding in cholate extract from dog striata was certainly of dopaminergic nature; first butyro-

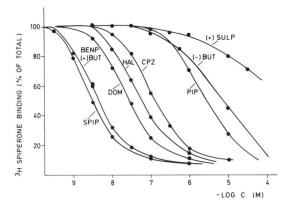

FIG. 1. Drug displacement of various compounds in ^{3}H-spiperone binding using cholate extract from dog striata. Spip, spiperone; Benp, benperidol; Dom, domperidone; Hal, haloperidol; CPZ, chlorpromazine; Pip, pipamperone; Sulp, sulpiride (cf. ref. 16).

phenones without spirodecanone moiety like benperidol and halo-peridol competed at nanomolar concentrations whereas pipam-perone, a serotonin antagonist, was active in the micromolar range. In our earlier experiments where only spirodecanone sites were extracted, benperidol was 3,800 times less active in soluble extracts than in membrane preparations. Table 2 clearly shows the different IC_{50}-values for binding sites of dopamin-ergic and serotonergic nature; three compounds, domperidone, pipamperone and a tetralin derivative are particularly useful perhaps even essential to differentiate both receptor sites. Pipamperone is a potent serotonin antagonist; the opposite is true for domperidone. Finally, the tetralin derivative is an agonist much more selective for dopamine than serotonin recep-tors. Recently, serotonin S_2 receptors were solubilized with CHAPS in a higher yield (40 %) than using lysolecithin (5 %) (35). Table 2 shows that both dopamine and serotonin receptors display pronounced differences in their pharmacological proper-ties independently of the detergent used for the solubilization procedure. The compounds listed in Table 2 represent the minimal number of drugs which are required to assess the dopaminergic nature of the binding sites.

Even if ^{3}H-spiperone can label membrane-bound serotonergic receptors (10 to 20 %) in the striatum, it is without conse-quence for the solubilization of dopamine receptors because serotonergic receptors are not solubilized by digitonin.

As previously reported in detail (4, 7, 12, 16, 29, 32) there were very good correlations between the IC_{50}-values obtained in solubilized and membrane preparations and even the ED_{50}-values in various pharmacological tests.

TABLE 2.   Drug potency for dopamine D_2 and serotonin S_2
receptors solubilized from striatum and cortex
of rat and human brain

Drug	IC_{50} (nM)			
	^3H-spiperone binding striatum (D_2)		^3H-ketanserin binding cortex (S_2)	
	Cholate		CHAPS	Lysolecithin
	Rat[a]	Human[a]	Rat[b]	Human[c]
Spiperone	1.8	3	3.8	7.1
Benperidol	3.8	5	–	–
(+)Butaclamol	7.6	5.1	13.8	42.2
Domperidone	20	22	1,320	247
2-(N,N-dipropyl)-amino-5,6-di-hydroxytetralin	575	575	224,000	66,800
Pipamperone	2,510	3,020	14.2	5.6
(–)Butaclamol	17,800	7,943	30,000	26,600

[a] values taken from ref. (32); [b] from (35) and [c] from (25).

Since the regional distribution of dopamine receptors in the brain is restricted to dopaminergic areas like caudate nucleus, olfactory tubercle and nucleus accumbens, it is often useful to perform the solubilization from cerebellum, for instance, which is devoid of dopamine receptors; this represents blank tissue, which is of value throughout the solubilization and the subsequent purification procedures.

PHOTOAFFINITY

The solubilization of a receptor consists of converting it from a complex membrane system into a relatively simple state; it is not a goal in itself but a prerequisite step to purify the receptor protein and to analyse its structure. Six years after the first report on the solubilization of high affinity dopamine receptors (7) one may be asked why dopamine receptors have not yet been obtained in a purified form. The reasons for this are far from clear but one may assume that practically all the attempts to purify the receptor protein through conventional techniques led to certain structural changes of the receptor site or its micelle in a way that it became undetectable in the binding assay; this was the case when using gel filtration techniques, affinity chromatography and even sedimentation gradient centrifugation.

^3H-Spiperone binding sites from soluble extracts from striata were reported to bind to wheat germ agglutinin agarose (5) or to concana valin A sepharose (29). However, the number of sites eluted from the column was very small and they were not clearly characterized as dopamine receptors. In fact, the binding activity is considerably, often even completely reduced, when a soluble extract is passed through any gel filtration columns. Similarly, dopamine receptors were only detectable after centrifugation in sedimentation gradients when high sucrose concentrations (20 to 30 %) were used to make the gradient; in such conditions the migration of protein only occurred over a short distance from the top of the gradient. Apparently something is lost when separation techniques are used to isolate the receptor protein.

Affinity chromatography appeared to be the method of choice; here again the results were negative. In our laboratory, Walter Wouters (30) synthesized fifteen different affinity gels with several ligands and different hydrophilic and hydrophobic arm spacers: dopamine receptors were found to bind to most of these gels but there was no detectable binding after elution.

After having had these problems one more approach remained, the photoaffinity. As shown in Fig. 2 two different probes were developed to label covalently dopamine receptors.

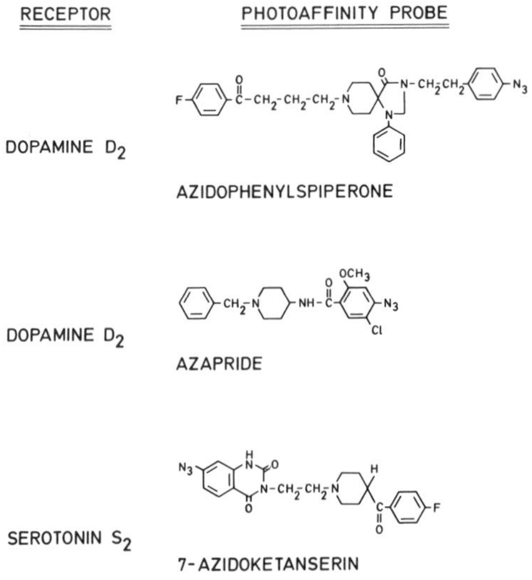

FIG. 2. Chemical structure of photoaffinity probes for dopamine D_2 and serotonin S_2 receptors

Azapride, an azido derivative of clebopride, behaved as a very selective dopamine antagonist and blocked irreversibly dopamine receptors from human (31) and rat (24, 33) striatum after irradiation with ultraviolet light. The irradiation-induced inactivation by azapride was prevented by dopamine antagonists and

TABLE 3. Binding affinity of photoaffinity probes and parent compound on dopamine D_2, serotonin S_2 and histamine H_1 receptors

	Affinity (nM)		
	[3H]-Spiperone (D_2) Kd	[3H]-Ketanserin (S_2) IC$_{50}$	[3H]-Pyrilamine (H_1) IC$_{50}$
Azidophenylethylspiperone (N$_3$-NAPS)	1.6	–	
Spiperone	0.25	–	
	IC$_{50}$		
Azapride	480	–	
Clebopride	42	–	
7-Azidoketanserin	–	2.9	1.2
Ketanserin	–	1.3	18.6

Values taken from ref. (1, 33, 36).

remained unchanged in the presence of scavenger p-amino benzoic acid indicating a true photoaffinity mechanism (24). However, as shown in Table 3, the compound does not reveal high affinity properties for dopamine receptors; this represents a serious drawback for its use at nanomolar concentrations in the labelled form.

Another photoaffinity probe, N_3-NAPS (1) was developed by starting from a potent spiperone analogue, the N-(p-aminophenethyl)spiperone (2). Table 3 shows that the azide derivative of this compound binds to dopamine receptors with high affinity. Recently it has been obtained in a radioiodinated form which was successfully used to identify a dopamine receptor subunit from crude membrane preparations (1). The molecular structure of dopamine receptors can be now completely dismantled. It is noteworthy that the photoaffinity approach seems only feasible when the probe keeps high affinity properties; it was the case for the spiperone derivative but also for the azidoketanserin which labels serotonin S_2 receptors as well as histamine H_1 sites (34, 36).

MOLECULAR CHARACTERIZATION

One of the first physical parameters that one wants to know about a receptor is its molecular size. Numerous methods are currently used to estimate the molecular weight of protein in solution; they are essentially based on sedimentation equilibrium in sucrose gradient, gel filtration and SDS gel electrophoresis. However, most of these methods are not devoid of major drawbacks which Barnard (3) has critically discussed taking as an example the nicotinic receptor. The data obtained from sedimentation gradient and gel filtration are mostly perturbed by an extensive binding of solubilizing detergent to the protein. By contrast, SDS electrophoresis is not affected by detergent. Another approach consists of high-energy radiation inactivation analysis whereby the size of a receptor can, in principle, be determined in the membrane-bound state.

The dopamine receptor is an intrinsic protein with an isoelectric point (pI-value) of 5.0 (21) which indicates that the receptor has a net negative charge at physiological pH. Since the determination of the molecular weight of intrinsic protein by means of sedimentation gradient remains approximate, it is not surprising that numerous different Svedberg values ($S_{20}W$) were reported for dopamine receptors. Table 4 shows the S-values, the estimated molecular weight and the Stoke radius of dopamine receptors from different species with various detergents. The sedimentation coefficient seems to be dependent not only in the nature of detergent but also on the presence or absence of salt or detergent in the gradient. For instance, when KCl was added to the sucrose gradient, the S-value was generally lower than in its absence; the reasons for this are not clear but a phenomenon of aggregation in the absence of

TABLE 4.   Molecular parameters of dopamine receptors

Source	Method	Sedimentation coefficient S	Molecular weight K	Stokes Radius nm	Reference
Dog	digitonin sucrose gradient	~ 12	200-300	–	(7)
	digitonin sucrose gradient + KCl	9	150-200	–	(16)
	digitonin sucrose gradient + Triton X-100	5.5	136	–	(21)
	gel filtration	–	–	5.8	(21)
	cholate/salt sucrose gradient + KCl	12	200-300	–	(32)
	gel filtration	–	–	5.65	(32)
	lysophosphatidylcholine				
	sucrose gradient	12.6	200-300	–	(29)
	sucrose gradient + KCl	9	150-200	–	(29)
	radiation inactivation	–	123	–	(22)
Human	cholate/salt sucrose gradient + KCl	2.5	60	–	(32)
	gel filtration	–	–	3.42	(32)
	radiation inactivation	–	123	–	(22)
Bovine	digitonin sucrose gradient	11.4	–	–	(29)
	gel filtration	–	–	8.0	(29)
	lysophosphatidylcholine				
	sucrose gradient	11.9	–	–	(29)
	gel filtration	–	150-200	–	(19)
	cholate/salt sucrose gradient	6	–	–	(29)
	gel filtration	–	–	6.6	(29)
	radiation inactivation	–	110 and 1,500	–	(11)
Rat	cholate/salt sucrose gradient + KCl	9	150-200	–	(32)
	SDS electrophoresis	–	94	–	(1)
	radiation inactivation	–	136	–	(23)

salt remains a plausible explanation. A sedimentation coefficient of 9 S was repeatedly found; this corresponds to a molecular weight of 150 to 200,000. Such a value is only slightly higher than that obtained by radiation inactivation. Values lower than 150 kilodalton were also reported, one from sedimentation gradient and another from SDS gel electrophoresis. A molecular weight of 60,000 dalton for human dopamine receptors is somewhat surprising; different explanations other than a real difference of size of dopamine receptors in human and in other animal species have been proposed (32). More interesting is the isolation of a Mr = 94,000 peptide by SDS electrophoresis which represents the ligand binding site of the dopamine D_2 receptor (1). As it is not known whether this peptide may itself represent a fragment of a larger polypeptide, a molecular weight for dopamine receptors higher than 94,000 dalton still remains possible. Gel electrophoresis does not in itself give information on an oligomeric molecular weight (3). In any case, N_3-NAPS certainly represents the most promising probe to explore in detail the molecular structure of dopamine receptors.

REFERENCES

1. Amlaiky, N., and Caron, M.G. (1985): J. Biol. Chem., 260: 1983-1986.
2. Amlaiky, N., Kilpatrick, B.F., and Caron, M.G. (1984): FEBS Lett., 176: 436-440.
3. Barnard, E.A. (1984): In: Investigation of Membrane-Located Receptors, edited by E. Reid, G.M.W. Cook, and D.J. Morré, pp. 59-82. Plenum Press, New York and London.
4. Davis, A., Madras, B., and Seeman, P. (1981): Eur. J. Pharmacol., 70: 321-329.
5. Goldstein, M., and Lew, J.Y. (1984): In: Catecholamines: Basic and Peripheral Mechanisms, edited by E. Usdin, A. Carlsson, A. Dahlström, and J. Engel, pp. 237-242. Alan R. Liss, New York.
6. Gorissen, H., and Laduron, P.M. (1978): Life Sci., 23: 575-580.
7. Gorissen, H., and Laduron, P.M. (1979): Nature, 279: 243-249.
8. Gorissen, H., Ilien, B., Aerts, G., and Laduron, P. (1980): FEBS Lett., 121: 133-138.
9. Hyttel, J. (1981): Life Sci., 28: 563-569.
10. Kebabian, J.W., and Calne, D.B. (1979): Nature, 277: 93-96.
11. Kuno, T., and Tanaka, C. (1983): Biochem. Biophys. Res. Commun., 117: 65-70.
12. Laduron, P. (1980): Trends Pharmacol. Sci., 1: 471-474.
13. Laduron, P.M. (1981): In: Apomorphine and Other Dopaminomimetics, edited by G.L. Gessa, and G.U. Corsini, pp. 95-103. Raven Press, New York.
14. Laduron, P.M. (1983): In: Dopamine Receptors, edited by C. Kaiser, and J.W. Kebabian, pp. 22-28. ACS Symposium Series 224, American Chemical Society, Washington.

15. Laduron, P.M., and Ilien, B. (1982): Biochem. Pharmacol., 31: 2145-2152.
16. Laduron, P.M., and Wouters, W. (1984): In: Catecholamines: Basic and Peripheral Mechanisms, edited by E. Usdin, A. Carlsson, A. Dahlström, and J. Engel, pp. 251-258. Alan R. Liss, New York.
17. Leff, S., and Creese, I. (1982): Biochem. Biophys. Res. Commun., 108: 1150-1157.
18. Leff, S.E., and Creese, I. (1983): Trends Pharmacol. Sci., 4: 463-466.
19. Lerner, M.H., Rosengarten, H., and Friedhoff, A.J. (1981): Life Sci., 29: 2367-2373.
20. Leysen, J.E. (1984): In: Advances in Human Psychopharmacology, edited by G.D. Burrows, and J. Werry, Vol. 3, pp. 315-356. JAI Press, Greenwich, Connecticut.
21. Lilly, L., Davis, A., Fraser, C.M., Seeman, P., and Venter, J.C. (1985): Neurochem. Int., 7: 363-368.
22. Lilly, L., Fraser, C.M., Jung, C., Seeman, P., and Venter, J.C. (1983): Mol. Pharmacol., 24: 10-14.
23. Nielsen, M., Klimek, V., and Hyttel, J. (1984): Life Sci., 35: 325-332.
24. Niznik, H.B., Guan, J.H., Neumeyer, J.L., and Seeman, P. (1984): Eur. J. Pharmacol., 104: 389-390.
25. Schotte, A., Maloteaux, J.M., and Laduron, P.M. (1984): Eur. J. Pharmacol., 100: 329-333.
26. Seeman, P. (1980): Pharmacol. Rev., 32: 229-313.
27. Seeman, P., Ulpian, C., Grigoriadis, D., Pri-Bar, I., and Buchman, O. (1985): Biochem. Pharmacol., 34: 151-154.
28. Stoof, J.C., and Kebabian, J.W. (1984): Life Sci., 35: 2281-2296.
29. Strange, P.G., Abbott, W.M., and Wheatley, M. (1984): In: Catecholamines: Basic and Peripheral Mechanisms, edited by E. Usdin, A. Carlsson, A. Dahlström, and J. Engel, pp. 251-258. Alan R. Liss, New York.
30. Wouters, W. (1985): Towards The Molecular Characterization of Dopamine D_2 and Serotonin S_2 Receptors. Solubilization and Photoaffinity Probes. Thesis, University of Antwerp.
31. Wouters, W., Van Dun, J., and Laduron, P.M. (1984): Biochem. Pharmacol., 33: 3517-3520.
32. Wouters, W., Van Dun, J., and Laduron, P.M. (1984): Biochem. Pharmacol., 33: 4039-4044.
33. Wouters, W., Van Dun, J., and Laduron, P.M. (1984): Eur. J. Biochem., 145: 273-278.
34. Wouters, W., Van Dun, J., Leysen, J.E., and Laduron, P.M. (1985): Eur. J. Pharmacol., 107: 399-400.
35. Wouters, W., Van Dun, J., Leysen, J.E., and Laduron, P.M. (1985): Eur. J. Pharmacol., 115: 1-9.
36. Wouters, W., Van Dun, J., Leysen, J.E., and Laduron, P.M. (1985): FEBS Lett., 182: 291-296.

Neurotransmitter Interactions in the Basal Ganglia, edited by M. Sandler et al.
Raven Press, New York © 1987.

MOLECULAR GENETICS : OUTLOOK IN PHARMACOLOGY AND CLINICAL INVESTIGATIONS.

J. Mallet, S. Berrard, F. Blanot, C. Boni, M. Buda*,
N. Faucon Biguet, B. Grima, Ph. Horellou, J.-F. Julien,
A. Lamouroux, J. Powell and T. Rhyner.

Laboratoire de Neurobiologie Cellulaire et Moléculaire,
Département de Génétique Moléculaire, Centre National de la
Recherche Scientifique, F - 91190 Gif-sur-Yvette, France.
* Institut National de la Santé et de la Recherche Médicale,
U.171, Hôpital Sainte-Eugénie, F-69230 Saint-Genis Laval,
France

INTRODUCTION

Molecular genetics has now become an integral part of biochemical research both fundamental and applied. The regulation of gene expression can now be analysed at the molecular level. A gene from any species can in principle be expressed in any cell line. This approach should facilitate the dissection of systems such as neurotransmitter metabolism, receptors and their transducing machinery. More particularly, the study of human genes should allow the development of model systems which should be most fruitful in the design and testing of new drugs. Many diseases have a genetic component and are therefore amenable to a molecular genetic analysis which should lead not only to improved diagnosis but also to a better understanding of the physiopathology and ultimately to a more rational therapy.

To illustrate these potentialities we will mostly refer to our work on tyrosine hydroxylase. This enzyme is the rate limiting enzyme in the synthesis of catecholamines. Interestingly, the regulation of its expression is under developmental control (27) and its synthesis can be induced <u>in vivo</u> by nerve stimulation (39, 44) or by treatment with <u>reserpine</u> (38, 34) or steroids (32). Also multiple kinase activities may be involved in the short-term regulation of catecholamine biosynthesis by afferent activity (32, 15).

This new molecular genetic methodology should also allow the identification of new proteins which play an important role in brain function but are present in too small amount to be isolated by conventional techniques. We describe here a technique which allows the detection and characterisation of such proteins.

A MOLECULAR GENETIC APPROACH TO THE STUDY OF TYROSINE HYDROXYLASE (TH)

Determination of the complete TH amino-acid sequence

The PC12 cell line which is derived from a rat pheochromo-cytoma tumor contains a relatively high level of TH enzyme. Molecular cloning starting from PC12 mRNA allowed us to isolate a cDNA containing the entire sequence of TH mRNA from which we could deduce the complete amino-acid sequence of the enzyme (26, 12) (Fig. 1).

A wealth of information can be obtained from the analysis of the amino-acid sequence. Taking into account available biochemical data (42) we could then infer that the active site is located in the C-terminal part of the enzyme (12). Three serine residues which are good candidates for phosphorylation (36, 24) are located in the N-terminal domain at position 19, 40 and 153. TH appears then to be composed of two distinct domains : one that performs the enzymatic reaction and another that modulates it.

The cDNA containing the complete coding sequence of rat TH mRNA was subcloned into a vector that contains the specific promoter of Salmonella typhimurium phage SP6. Since the corresponding RNA polymerase efficiently initiates transcription only at SP6 phage promoters, microgram amounts of RNA could be produced. In the reticulocyte lysate translation system or after microinjection into frog oocytes, this mRNA directs the synthesis of a protein which comigrates with native PC12 TH. Furthermore, the TH protein produced in the oocyte has the ability to promote the synthesis of dopa from tyrosine (Horellou et al., in preparation). The post-translationnal modifications which modulate the activity of the enzyme can now be analysed and those amino acid residues that are essential for TH activity and regulation can be identified by mutagenesis studies.

Initial Northern blot experiments (11) indicated that rat cDNA clones recognize human TH mRNA purified from a human pheochromocytoma tumor. A cDNA library was generated from this tissue and the corresponding human TH cDNA clones were detected with the rat probe. The longest clone containing 1526 bp was sequenced. The alignment of the amino acid sequence with that of the rat is shown in Fig. 1. On the same figure is also shown the homology between TH and phenylalanine hydroxylase (PH). Clearly TH and PH possess a high degree of homology in their central and carboxyl terminus regions. These findings are not surprising considering that both enzymes are mixed-function oxidases and share many characteristic biochemical and immunological properties (21, 9, 8).

It will be of interest to compare the sequences of TH and PH with that of tryptophan hydroxylase which also utilizes

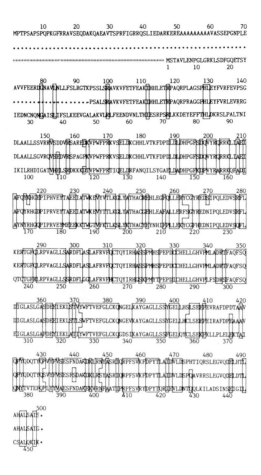

FIG.1. Alignment of the amino acid sequence of rat
TH (top), a fragment of human TH (middle), and human
phenylalanine hydroxylase (PH, bottom). The sequences
for rat TH and human PH have been taken from references 12 and 24, respectively. The one-letter amino acid
notation is used. Identical residues between the three
sequences are boxed.

molecular oxygen to oxidize simultaneously an aromatic acid substrate and tetrahydrobiopterin (21).

Transcriptional regulation of TH gene expression

Stimulations such as cold stress, or the administration of reserpine cause an increase of TH activity and the effect lasts as long as 3 weeks. Interruption of the afferent nerves to the adrenals or superior cervical ganglia abolished the effect which has, therefore, been referred to as trans-synaptic induction. The increase in TH activity that occurs in adrenal medulla and locus coeruleus following administration of reserpine has been shown by immunoprecipitation studies to result from an increase in the amount of TH and not from an activation of pre-existing enzyme molecules (34). Reserpine acts by interfering with the transport of catecholamines into the storage vesicles and provides a convenient model to study the mechanism of induction of this enzyme (6,7).

Rats have been injected with a single dose of reserpine and changes in mRNA and enzyme activity were analysed at various times in locus coeruleus, substantia nigra and adrenals (7). A quantitative and sensitive Northern blot procedure was first developed which allowed the analysis of TH mRNA in those structures from a single rat (7). Many samples can be processed simultaneously and the method is suitable for routine pharmacological tests.

The time course analysis is shown in Fig. 2. These data, as well as those obtained from actinomycin D experiments (31) suggest that the increase in enzyme activity in adrenals and locus coeruleus reflects an enhanced transcription of the TH gene. No effect was observed in substantia nigra in agreement with the previous work of Reis et al. (34).

Surprisingly, Fig. 2 also indicates that both in the adrenals and locus coeruleus, the maximal relative increase of TH mRNA is much higher than that of enzyme activity. Also, TH mRNA levels decrease sharply after day 2, suggesting that the available pool of TH mRNA has not been efficiently processed to increase enzyme activity. The decay profiles of TH mRNA and enzyme activity are, however, quite different in adrenals and locus coeruleus. Clearly, reserpine elicits a much longer lasting effect in the brain nuclei than in the peripheral catecholaminergic cells. In the adrenals, TH mRNA level has almost returned to the initial value at day 4, whereas it is still 3-fold higher in the locus coeruleus. In fact, in this latter structure, after day 4 both TH mRNA and enzyme levels decline slowly. The effect of the drug is still significant at day 18, confirming earlier TH activity studies by Zigmond (45). At this stage, it is attractive to speculate that the difference in the amplitude of the effects observed after day 4, between locus coeruleus and adrenals, results from a

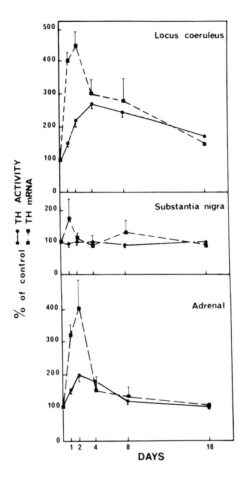

FIG. 2.   Time course of changes in TH mRNA and TH
activity in   the locus coeruleus, substantia nigra
and adrenals of rats following administration of a
single dose of reserpine. The results are expressed
as percentage of control rats injected with the
appropriate vehicle and sacrificed at the same time.
Results of TH activity and TH mRNA are means ± SEM
of 3 to 5 independent experiments.

difference in the stability of the TH mRNA. Experiments on
isolated nuclei should allow us to test this hypothesis.
Clearly the events linking the increase in neural activity and
long lasting changes in neuronal properties have only begun to
be explored.

Interestingly, this study also revealed that, in the adrenal
medulla where the enzyme is. not transported, both the amount
of TH mRNA per cell and the ratio of TH mRNA to enzyme activity are lower than in the catecholaminergic cells of the brain
(7).

Because of the great heterogeneity of nervous tissue, it is
desirable that specific mRNA hybridizations be detected at the
cellular level. In situ hybridization histochemistry is now
being developed in various laboratories and in a first series
of experiments we could recently detect TH mRNA in the substantia nigra and locus coeruleus of the rat brain (A. Berod et
al, manuscript in preparation).

Analysis of the rat TH gene

A rat genomic library was constructed using a cosmid vector
that contains, as a dominant selectable eukaryotic marker, the
neomycin resistance gene under the control of the Herpes
Simplex virus thymidine kinase promoter sequences (13). From
the initial screening of 400,000 recombinant clones, two
clones were isolated which hybridised positively with the rat
cDNA probe. The sequences contained in these two clones span
approximately 55 kb of chromosomal DNA, and clone cosTH-1 was
shown to contain the complete TH gene which is about 12 kb.

In a first series of experiments aimed at analyzing the
functional role of sequences preceding the coding portion of
the TH gene, CosTH-1 was introduced by the calcium phosphate
precipitate method (11) into mouse neuroblastoma and a hamster
glial cell line that does not produce detectable levels of TH
mRNA. In both instances, neomycin resistant clones were
visible after 2 to 3 weeks. Several clones were isolated and
tested for the presence of TH mRNA. About half of the selected
clones expressed an mRNA species that was recognized by the TH
probe. On Northern blots, the mRNA bands were identical in
size with that of mRNA from PC12 cells. The relative abundance
of this hybridising species with respect to the total amount
of total mRNA, was variable in different clones and represented, in one glial cell transformant, about one fifth the
amount of TH mRNA present in PC12 cells. S1 mapping experiments are now being conducted to confirm that transformants
express mRNA coding for TH, which is identical to that of TH
producing cells. The expression of TH protein was first tested
with a TH antibody. A positive reaction could only be observed
with the transformed glial cell line that produced the highest
amount of TH-like mRNA. The corresponding enzyme activity

could, however, not be detected. Clearly, DNA–mediated gene transfer represents also a powerful approach to dissect out the events necessary for the expression of enzymatically active TH molecules, and the above results open the way to a detailed analysis of sequences required for TH gene transcription.

Human genetics of TH

The human TH gene was first assigned to chromosome 11 by the analysis of DNA from a panel of human – mouse cell hybrids using the human cDNA probe (33). Analysis of silver grain distribution, following in situ hybridization with the same probe on both male and female chromosome preparations, confirmed the assignment and provided a regional localization to 11p15 (5).

In view of the strong homology between TH and PH, it is of interest to note that PH has been localized to the long arm of chromosome 12 (28). Similarly, other homologous genes, such as insulin-like growth factors I and II, have been assigned to the short arm of chromosome 11 and to the long arm of chromosome 12, respectively (10). These findings are at first surprising, but are not irrational. They add further weight to the speculation, originally based on similarities of morphology and banding pattern, that chromosomes 11 and 12 result from an ancient tetraploidisation, and support the suggestion by Brissenden et al. (3) that the relative order of loci on the two chromosomes may have been disrupted by a pericentric inversion.

Digestion of human cellular DNA with the restriction endonuclease Eco RI revealed a high frequency restriction fragment length polymorphism (RFLP) which constitutes a suitable marker for future linkage studies involving the TH gene. More particularly, there is now little doubt that psychiatric disorders exhibit familial segregation. Depression is generally related to a deficiency of catecholamine (usually norepinephrine) at functionally important central adrenergic receptors. Mania and schizophrenia, on the other hand, are thought to result from an excess of catecholamines, more particularly dopamine in the latter case. It is then of importance to establish whether TH gene markers segregate with these diseases in large reference families where homogeneity and high penetrance of the trait has been carefully established.

Other affective disorders such as phobias and autism exhibit genetic susceptibility and are also likely to result from a defect in neurotransmission. Relevant probes coding for enzymes, peptides and receptors are becoming available at an increasing pace and should prove in some instances useful to localize susceptibility loci which might reside in the coding region of a candidate gene or most probably in the region controlling its expression.

Whenever this approach, which is referred to as the "best guess" strategy is proved negative, the corresponding candidate gene will be at least eliminated. In those instances, the availability of a collection of genomic DNA from reference families carrying a particular trait, leaves the possibility of applying the "linkage" approach using random DNA markers. This strategy has been particularly successful in the case of Huntington's disease (14). In principle, the uncovering of reasonably closely linked DNA markers will ultimately result in the identification of the susceptibility locus and primary gene defect. A molecular understanding of the physiopathology of the disease should then follow, opening new avenues for pharmacological research. Most probably, this knowledge will also be of great value to analyse closely related diseases which occur sporadically or in which the genetic predisposition is ill-defined. A case in point concerns Alzheimer disease. Only a few examples have been found, up until now, to segregate in families in a dominant autosomal manner. The origin of the disease is unknown and no significant clinical or neuropathological differences between the sporadic and familial forms have been revealed. This socio-economically important illness is now the focus of much attention and it is very likely that the genetic linkage method and family studies will bring new and decisive information.

A NOVEL APPROACH TO EXPLORE THE MOLECULAR BASIS OF BRAIN FUNCTION

The nervous system of higher vertebrates is characterized by a wide anatomical and functional diversity. To generate such a complexity, a high proportion of the genome is transcribed in the brain, relative to any other peripheral organ (20, 4). According to these reports, as many as 150,000 genes are expressed in this tissue and about 40 % of the mRNAs represent specific transcripts (30). Consequently, protein chemistry of the nervous system has been hampered by the low concentration of most individual species. Only a few dozen brain specific proteins have so far been purified to homogeneity. Monoclonal antibody technology has proved useful for their identification in some instances (22, 41), but the selection of the clones of interest is often a tedious task.

The recent advances of molecular genetics provide a powerful approach to identify and thereafter to purify relevant proteins. Along this line, Milner and Sutcliffe (30) have recently generated a cDNA library of adult rat poly(A)+mRNA and could select, by Northern blot analysis, clones corresponding to mRNAs which are specifically expressed in brain.

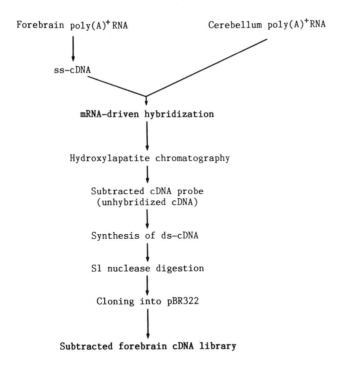

FIG. 3.   Scheme for the cloning of subtracted cDNA.

An alternative strategy is based on the differential screening of recombinant colonies generated from a given tissue with various cDNA probes of different specificity. This method which is often referred to as "Plus and minus screening" was successfully applied in our laboratory in isolating TH cDNA clones (26). Taking into account that TH is a tissue specific protein, a cDNA library derived from PC12 cells was screened with cDNA probes generated from the same cells and from liver. Only 10 % of the clones exhibited the expected pattern of hybridization which considerably facilitated the selection process (26). A 5-fold difference in mRNA level can be detected with this procedure which permits the detection of mRNA expressed at a level as low as 0.01 % (35). This sensitivity is nevertheless not sufficient to identify many important brain mRNAs whose abundance is much lower.

The differential screening method could be however greatly improved through the use of subtracted probes, both for generating cDNA libraries and for screening them. The principle of this procedure resides in specific cDNA-mRNA hybridizations followed by purification of the unhybridized cDNA by hydroxylapatite chromatography. Following the scheme described in Figure 3, we have constructed a forebrain cDNA library from which cerebellum sequences have been largely removed. This library was constructed as a first step toward our objective of determining whether specific transcripts can be identified that are induced by sleep deprivation. Subtractions were performed with cerebellum because, in contrast to the profound degree of integrative function of the forebrain, this tissue is mostly involved in lower functions such as planning, initiation and control of movement (1). The cell composition and cytoarchitectonic organization of these two structures also differ greatly, but nevertheless they have an almost analogous complexity as shown by liquid hybridization (20). These differences must therefore arise from the presence of a set of different transcripts expressed at low levels in the two tissues.

The experimental details of the procedure are described in reference (34b). About 90 % by weight of the cDNAs derived from forebrain were eliminated after hybridization to cerebellum poly(A)+RNA. The potentialities of this method is examplified in Figure 4 which represents a set of 200 clones (among 7000) of the subtracted library which have been triplicated and screened with cDNA probes generated from cerebral cortex, brainstem, hippocampus and subtracted with cerebellum poly(A)+RNA. Regional distribution was clearly observed. Although some clones were detected using all three probes, most of them hybridized with only one (one arrow) or two (two arrows) of these cDNA populations. A total of 10 clones were selectively expressed in only one of these areas. Interestingly, these regionally distributed clones were not revealed with unsubtracted probes.

Clearly, as previously reported (40, 37, 22, 16) the use of absorbed probes greatly enhances the sensitivity of the screening procedures. A quantitative assessment was performed by adding previously characterized TH cDNA clones (26) on the filters that were analysed with subtracted probes from various brain regions. The brainstem probe recognized TH clones, and no hybridization was observed with the hippocampus probe, confirming the distribution of TH neurones in rat brain (17, 18). Interestingly, under careful inspection, TH clones also exhibited a positive signal with the cerebral cortex probe, relative to the adjacent control clones. This result was unexpected, although a few dopaminergic cells have been identified in this structure in the primate (23). The presence of TH mRNA was verified by Northern blot analysis (34b) and its abundance was estimated to be of the order of 0.0001%. This value represents the extreme sensitivity limit of the colony hybridization method using subtracted probes and corresponds to a potential 50-fold improvement over the conventional techniques. Very low amounts of TH mRNA could also be detected in hippocampus by Northern blot analysis.

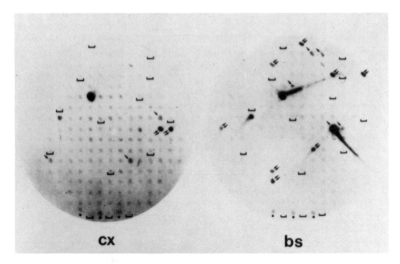

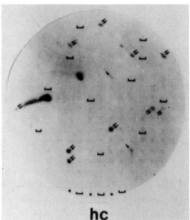

FIG. 4. Detection by colony hybridization of clones characteristic to various areas of the brain. Two hundred clones chosen at random from the subtracted forebrain library have been placed on the three filters. The marked areas (. , bottom of the filters) correspond to TH cDNA clones (pTH 51). The cDNA probes were subtracted with cerebellum poly(A)+RNA prior to filter hybridization. a: cerebral cortex probe (6 x 10 c.p.m./ml). b: brainstem probe (9 x 10^5 c.p.m./ml). c: hippocampus probe (9 x 10^5 c.p.m./m l). Exposure time of the autoradiograms was 5 days.

Further investigation is needed to understand the functional significance of this residual expression.

The use of subtracted probes both to construct cDNA libraries and to screen them represents an efficient procedure to identify mRNAs expressed at very low levels. Careful screening requires that the colonies be arranged manually on the filters and this imposes a limit upon the number of clones which can be analysed. The "enrichment" of the library greatly reduces the number of clones to be screened and facilitates the identification of clones which are specific to various parts of the brain. In contrast, dealing with a corresponding unsubtracted cDNA population would be an enormous task.

The applications of this methodology are numerous and should allow the identification of clones corresponding to functionally important proteins, such as neurotransmitter-synthesising enzymes, receptors, and ionic channels. It should also facilitate the study of transcripts which are stage- or tissue-specific, or whose expression in mature brain is physiologically or pharmacologically modulated. Subtracted libraries from individual structures may also be generated to facilitate identification of these characteristic transcripts. However, many brain functions are not restricted or have not been attributed to a given area, and in many instances, it will therefore be necessary to screen a forebrain library with probes generated from various structures. The isolation of specific sequences permits access to the protein itself for the study of its structure, function and regulation. Furthermore, the use of an antibody, combined with in situ hybridizations, can reveal important properties of the protein, with respect to its transport along nerve fibers, secretion and membrane insertion. By such means, it may be hoped that many important proteins will be uncovered that would not have been accessible by conventional biochemical techniques. Some of them will proved to be important new targets for pharmacological research.

Acknowledgements

We wish to thank Ph. Vernier for critical reading of the manuscript, and D. Samolyk, G. Peudevin and D. Rouxel for efficient technical assistance. This work was supported by grants from the Centre National de la Recherche Scientifique, the Fondation pour la Recherche Médicale Française, the Association pour la Recherche sur le Cancer and Rhône-Poulenc Santé.

References

1. Allen, G.I., and Tsukahara, N. (1974): Physiol. Rev. 54: 957–1006.
2. Barnstable, C.J. (1980): Nature (London) 286:231–235.
3. Brissenden, J.E., Ullrich, A. and Franke, U. (1984): Nature 310:781–784.
4. Chikaraishi, D.M. (1979): Biochemistry 18:3249–3256.

5. Craig, S.P., Buckle, V.J., Lamouroux, A., Mallet, J. and Craig, I.W. Cytogenet. Cell Genet. (in press).
6. Faucon Biguet, N., Boni, C., Buda, M., Grima, B., Julien, J.F., Lamouroux, A. and Mallet, J. (1984): In: "Catecholamines", edited by E.Usdin, A. Carlsson, A. Dahlström and J. Engel,Part C, pp.211-218. A.R. Liss, New York.
7. Faucon Biguet, N., Buda, M., Lamouroux, A., Samolyk, D. and Mallet, J. (1986): EMBO J.   5:287-291.
8. Fisher, D.B. and Kaufman, S. (1972): J. Biol. Chem. 247:2250-2252.
9. Friedman, P.A., Lloyd T., and Kaufman, S. (1972): Mol. Pharmacol. 8:501-510.
10. Gera.d, P.S. and Grzeschik. K.H. (1984): Cytogenet. Cell Genet. 37:103-126.
11. Graham, F. L. and van der Eb, A.J. (1973): Virology 52: 456-467.
12. Grima, B., Lamouroux, A., Blanot, F., Faucon Biguet, N., and Mallet, J. (1985): Proc. Natl. Acad. Sci. USA, 82:617-621.
13. Grosveld, F.G., Lund, T., Murray, E.J., Mellor, A.L., Dahl. H.H.M. and Flavell, R.A. (1981): Nucleic Acids Res.,10:6715-6732.
14. Gusella, J.F., Tanzi, R.E., Anderson, M.A., Hobbs, W., Gibbons, K., Raschtchian, R., Gillam, T.C., Wallace, M.R., Wexler, N.S. and Conneally, P.M. (1984): Science 225:1320-1326.
15. Haycock, J.W., Bennett, W.F., George, R.J. and Waymire J.C. (1982): J.Biol.Chem., 257:13699-13703.
16. Hedrick, S.M., Cohen, D.I., Nielsen, E.A., Davis, M.M. (1984): Nature (London) 308:149-153.
17. Hökfelt, T., Johansson, O., Fuxe, K.,   Goldstein, M. and Park, D. (1976): Med. Biol. 54:427-453.
18. Hökfelt, T., Johansson, O., Fuxe, K., Goldstein, M., and Park, D. (1977): Med. Biol. 55:21-40.
19. Joh, T.H., Park, D.H. and Reis, D.J. (1978): Proc. Natl. Acad. Sci. USA, 75:4744-4748.
20. Kaplan, B.B., Schachter, B.S., Osterburg, H.H., de Vellis, J.S., and Finch, C.E. (1978) Biochemistry, 17: 5516-5523.
21. Kaufman, S. and Fisher, D.B. (1974): In: Molecular Mechanism of Oxygen Activation, edited by O., Hayaishi, pp. 285-368, Academic Press, New York.
22. Kavathas, P., Sukhatme, V.P., Herzenberg, L.A., and Parnes, J.P. (1984): Proc.Natl.Acad.Sci., USA.,81:7688-7692.
23. Köhler, C., Everitt, B.J., Pearson, J., and Goldstein, M. (1983) Neurosci. Lett. 37:161-166.
24. Krebs, E.L. and Beavo, J.A. (1979): Annu. Rev. Biochem. 48:923-959.
25. Kwok, S.C.M., Ledley, F.D., DiLella, A.G., Robson, K.J.H., and Woo, S.L.C. (1985): Biochemistry, 24:556-561.

26. Lamouroux, A., Faucon Biguet, N., Samolyk, D., Privat, A., Salomon, J.C., Pujol, J.F., and Mallet, J. (1982): Proc. Natl. Acad.Sci., USA., 79:3881-3885.
27. Le Douarin, N. (1980): Nature (London), 286:663-669.
28. Lidsky, A.S., Robson, K.J.H., Thirumalachary, C., Barker, P.E., Ruddle, F.H. and Woo, S.L.C. (1984): Am. J. Hum. Genet. 36:527-533.
29. Mestikawy, S.E.L., Glowinski, J. and Hamon, M. (1983): Nature (London) 302:830-832.
30. Milner, R.J., and Sutcliffe, J.G. (1983): Nucl. Acids Res., 11:5497-5520.
31. Mueller, R.A., Thoenen, H. and Axelrod J. (1969): Mol. Pharmacol. 5:463-469.
32. Otten, U. and Thoenen, H. (1977): J. Neurochem. 29: 69-75.
33. Powell, J.F., Boni, C., Lamouroux, A., Craig, I.W. and Mallet, J. (1984) Febs. Lett. 175:31-40.
34. Reis, D.J., Joh, T.H. and Ross, R.A. (1975): J.Pharmacol. Exp. Ther. 193: 775-784.
34b. Rhyner, T., Faucon Biguet, N., Berrard, S., Borbely, A.A. and Mallet, J. Nucl. Acids Res. (in press).
35. StJohn, T.P., and Davis, R.W. (1979): Cell 16:443-452.
36. Shenolikar, S. and Cohen, P. (1970): FEBS Lett. 86: 92-98.
37. Scott, M.R.D., Westphal, K-H., Rigby, P.W.J. 1983): Cell 34:557-567.
38. Thoenen, H., Mueller, R.A. and Axelrod, J. (1969): J.Pharmacol. Exp. Ther. 169:249-254.
39. Thoenen, H. (1974): Life Sci., 14:223-235.
40. Timberlake, W.E. (1980) : Dev. Biol. 78:497-510.
41. Trisler, G.D., Schneider, M.D., Nirenberg, M. (1981): Proc. Natl. Acad. Sci., USA 78:2145-2149.
42. Vigny, A. and Henry, J.P. (1981): J. Neurochem. 36: 483-489.
43. Vigny, A. and Henry, J.P. (1982): Biochem. Biophys. Res. Commun. 106:1-7.
44. Zigmond, R.E. and Chalazonitis, A. (1979): Brain. Res., 164:137-152.
45. Zigmond, R.E. (1979): J. Neurochem. 32:23-29.

Subject Index